W9-BEQ-547

THE
Runner's World
KNEE BOOK

Look for these and other books of interest from *Runner's World* and Collier Books

The Runner's World Knee Book
The Competitive Runner's Training Book
Running After Forty
Dance Aerobics
The Complete Stretching Book
Run Farther, Run Faster
Running to the Top
The Triathlon Training Book
The *Runner's World* Training Diary
Serious Cycling for Beginners
Cures for Common Running Injuries
Beginner's Racquetball
Complete Woman's Weight Training Guide

THE
Runner's World
KNEE BOOK

What Every Athlete Needs to Know about the Prevention and Treatment of Knee Problems

by Alan A. Halpern, M.D.

Illustrations by Judith Johnson

COLLIER BOOKS
Macmillan Publishing Company
New York

Collier Macmillan Publishers
London

Copyright ©1984
Anderson World Books, Inc.

All rights reserved. No part of this book may be reproduced or transmitted in any form or by any means, electronic or mechanical, including photocopying, recording or by any information storage and retrieval system, without permission in writing from the Publisher.

Macmillan Publishing Company
866 Third Avenue, New York, N.Y. 10022
Collier Macmillan Canada, Inc.

Library of Congress Cataloging in Publication Data

Halpern, Alan A.
  The Runner's world knee book.

  Includes index.
  1. Knee-Wounds and injuries. 2. Running—Accidents and injuries. I.
Runner's World. II. Title.
III. Title: Knee book.
RD561.H35   1985   617'.582044   84-15526
ISBN 0-02-547500-2
ISBN 0-02-014010-X (pbk.)

Drawings on page 58 and 131 are from *O'Connor's Testbook of Arthroscopic Surgery,* Heshmat Shahriaree, editor; J.B. Lippincott Company, 1984, with permission.

Macmillan books are available at special discounts for bulk purchases for sales promotions, premiums, fund-raising, or educational use. Special editions or book excerpts can also be created to specification. For details, contact:
Special Sales Director
Macmillan Publishing Company
866 Third Avenue
New York, New York 10022

First Collier Books Edition 1984

The Runner's World Knee Book is also published in a hardcover edition by Macmillan Publishing Company.

10 9 8 7 6 5 4 3 2 1

Printed in the United States of America

CONTENTS

This book is not intended as a substitute for medical advice of a physician. The reader should regularly consult a physician in matters relating to his or her health and particularly in respect to any symptoms that may require diagnosis or medical attention.

I wish to express my appreciation to Ms. Nancy Ehrle, who typed and edited the manuscript, to Professor David A. Winter of the University of Waterloo for his helpful comments, to Judith Johnson, who illustrated the book, and particularly to my wife, Judy.

The book is dedicated to my family, my love and inspiration.

1

INTRODUCING THE KNEE

The knee is the largest and one of the most complex joints in the body. It is particularly prone to injuries and arthritis. Some of our favorite activities such as skiing, football and running are responsible for thousands of knee injuries each year. In addition, many forms of arthritis affect the knee joint much more frequently and severely than other joints.

The current trend toward a more active population is placing greater demands on the knee. Sporting events, as well as running, are particularly stressful to a normal knee joint. Major advances in preventive medicine and treatment of many serious diseases now allow people to live longer, more active lives, placing greater stress on the weight-bearing joints for many more years.

Fortunately, new techniques and early diagnosis as well as more sophisticated rehabilitation practices have enabled physicians to treat injuries much more effectively. In many cases, prompt and effective treatment can prevent the development of serious instability and arthritis. Many people are able to return to vigorous, active lives instead of having their activities severely restricted due to incompletely treated knee injuries.

The purpose of this book is to give you a better understanding of the structure and function of the knee, the complex injuries that can occur, the nature of the medical and surgical treatments required for certain conditions and the rehabilitation necessary for recovery. My further purpose is to teach you habits and exercises which can protect your knee from injury.

2

ANATOMY OF THE KNEE

The knee is a complex joint which functions basically as a hinge while allowing rotation and gliding of one bone on another. There are actually two joints in the knee. The major weight-bearing joint is between the femur (thighbone) and the tibia (shinbone). There is also a smaller joint between the patella (kneecap) and the front of the femur.

During normal walking, forces of up to three times the body's weight are placed directly across the knee joint. A properly functioning knee depends not only on the joint surface itself but also on the capsule, tendons, ligaments and muscles surrounding the knee.

Bones of the Knee

The knee is composed of three bones: the femur, the tibia and the patella. The femur is the largest bone in the body, forming the hip joint at its upper end and the knee joint at its lower end. The tibia forms the lower end of the knee joint and has the ankle joint at its lower end. The patella forms the joint with the femur, allows the body to increase the effectiveness of its muscle power, and also serves to protect the front of the knee from direct injury. The fibula, the bone which runs parallel to the tibia, does not actually connect with the knee joint but has a separate small joint beneath it with the tibia.

The surface of the tibial joint is known as the tibial plateau. The

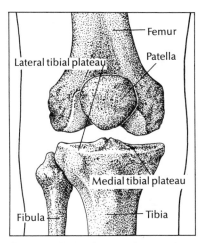

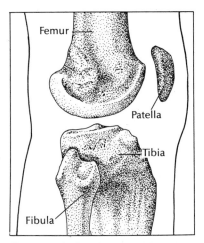

Bones of the knee—front view.
The knee is composed of three bones: the femur, the tibia and the patella.

Bones of the knee—side view.
The kneecap protects the knee from direct trauma and also increases the mechanical advantage of the quadriceps.

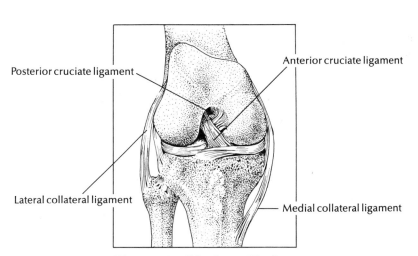

Ligaments of the knee. *The knee is supported by ligaments—the lateral collateral on the outside, the medial collateral on the inside and two cruciate ligaments in the middle.*

portion of the bone on the inside of the knee is known as the medial tibial plateau; and that on the outside is the lateral tibial plateau. The joint surface of the femur consists of two condyles (raised surfaces): the medial condyle and the lateral condyle. The space between them is known as the notch.

Ligaments of the Knee

Ligaments are structures which connect bones to other bones to stabilize the joints and help them support the body. There are four major ligaments in the knee.

The Medial Collateral Ligament. The medial collateral ligament runs on the inside of the knee between the femur and the tibia and prevents the knee from being stretched outward. This ligament has a deep portion which runs quite near the bone and also connects to the meniscus and has a more superficial portion which runs down the side of the bone. The medial collateral ligament is the most frequently injured ligament in the knee.

The Lateral Collateral Ligament. The lateral collateral ligament runs on the outside of the knee connecting the femur and the fibula and prevents the knee from being pushed inward. It is smaller than the medial collateral ligament and is injured less frequently.

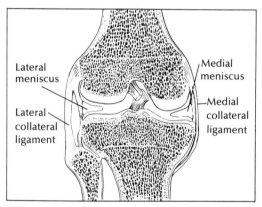

Cross section of the knee. *The menisci serve as shock absorbers for the knees; ligaments stabilize the knee.*

The Cruciate Ligaments. There are two ligaments called cruciates located in the middle of the knee. Both are vitally important. They are called "cruciate" because they cross. The anterior cruciate ligament prevents the knee from being pulled forward and stabilizes it from being pulled outward. The anterior cruciate ligament is fundamentally important for stabilization of the knee, particularly in competitive athletics. The average adult anterior cruciate ligament can withstand more than 200 pounds of force. Normal walking creates about 50 pounds of force, while jogging places a force of more than 150 pounds across the ligament. The posterior cruciate ligament crosses the anterior cruciate ligament and prevents the knee from being pushed backward. It is injured much less frequently than other ligaments.

Cartilages (The Menisci)

In addition to the cartilage at the end of the bone, the knee contains two crescent- or moon-shaped cartilages known as menisci.

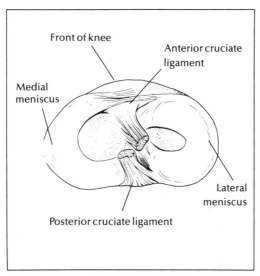

Cartilages of the knee. The knee contains two crescent-shaped cartilages called menisci, which serve as shock absorbers.

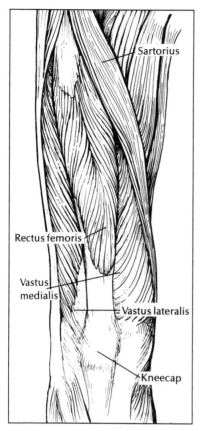

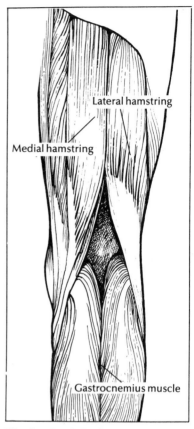

The quadriceps muscles. The quadriceps muscles straighten or extend the knee and run along the front of the femur.

The back of the knee (right leg). Two major muscle groups are responsible for bending the knee—the hamstrings, behind the thigh, and the gastrocnemius, on the back of the calf.

The medial meniscus is on the inside of the knee; the lateral meniscus on the outside. When functioning properly, these cartilages act as shock absorbers to protect joint surfaces from excessive wear. Between 50 and 60 percent of the body's weight is born by the meniscal cartilages. Meniscal cartilages are prone to injury in competitive athletics—knee surgery is frequently designed for treatment of meniscal tears.

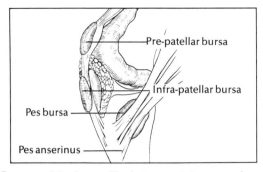

Bursae of the knee. *The knee contains many bursae where tendons rub across the bony surfaces.*

Muscles of the Knee

Numerous muscles are responsible for the proper functioning of the knee: the quadriceps, the hamstrings and the gastrocnemius. The quadriceps extends or straightens the knee, while the hamstrings bend or flex the joint. The quadriceps is actually a group of four muscles originating near the hip and running along the front of the femur. It consists of the rectus femoris, which runs down the middle; the vastus lateralis, which runs on the outside of the leg; the vastus medialis, which runs on the inside of the leg; and the vastus intermedius, which runs down the middle underneath the rectus femoris. The quadriceps is attached to the top of the kneecap, which is connected to the tibia by the patellar tendon. The vastus medialis muscle is particularly important for stabilizing the kneecap and is one of the earliest to atrophy when the knee is not properly exercised.

A group of muscles found behind the knee—the hamstrings—is responsible for bending or flexing the knee. There are two sets of hamstrings. The medial hamstrings, located on the inside of the knee, are composed of the semimembranosus, semitendinosis gracilis and the sartorius. The lateral hamstring is the biceps femoris muscle on the outside of the knee. The gastrocnemius muscle is connected to the femur behind the knee and aids in bending the knee. The other end of the gastrocnemius is connected to the Achilles tendon and is responsible for plantarflexing or pushing the ankle down. A small muscle behind the knee, the popliteus, runs toward the lateral aspect of the leg and helps to stabilize the knee.

A group of three muscles comes together on the inside of the knee at a tendon called the pes anserinus (so-called because it resembles a goose's foot). The muscles—the sartorius, gracilis and semitendinosus—are responsible for controlling some of the rotation of the knee.

The Iliotibial Tract

The iliotibial tract is a dense band of fibrous tissue found along the outside of the knee. The band originates by the hip where it is connected with the gluteus maximus and tensor fascia lata muscles. It is also connected with the outside of the femur and the front of the tibia. The band helps to stabilize the outside of the knee. On occasion, part of the iliotibial tract is used to replace damaged ligaments in the knee.

The Joint

The joint consists of opposing surfaces of a smooth, glistening substance called cartilage. When functioning at its best, cartilage allows stable. pain-free motion in the knee. The cartilage which covers the ends of bones is known as hyaline cartilage. It is a highly specialized tissue which serves not only as a shock absorber, but also as a low friction surface for motion. Cartilage consists of cells called chondrocytes surrounded by a network of collagen fibers imbedded in a gel-like substance composed of proteoglycans. Almost three fourths of the cartilage is composed of water. Collagen is a protein composed of amino acids arranged in a helix. Cartilage has no blood vessels and receives its nutrition from the joint (synovial) fluid.

The Capsule

The knee joint is surrounded by a capsule which keeps lubricating fluid in the joint and helps stabilize the knee. The posterior capsule is particularly important for providing this stability. A portion of this capsule just behind the medial collateral ligament has been named the posterior oblique ligament because of the strength of the fibers in this area. Tears of the anterior cruciate ligament are frequently associated with tears of this part of the

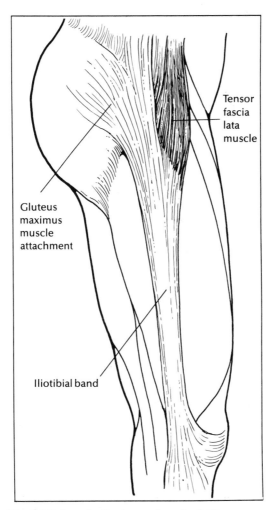

*Tensor
fascia
lata
muscle*

*Gluteus
maximus
muscle
attachment*

Iliotibial band

Iliotibial band. *A strong band of fibers runs
along the outside of the leg, attaching to the tibia
and sending some fibers to the kneecap.*

capsule. The back of the knee laterally contains a Y-shaped ligament called the arcuate, which stabilizes the knee during rotation.

The Synovium. The joint is lined by a very specialized cell layer called synovium. These cells are responsible for producing the joint or synovial fluid—essential for lubrication of the joint surfaces and nutrition of the cartilage. When inflammation occurs, the synovium produces excessive amounts of fluid leading to an effusion or "water on the knee."

3

WHAT CAN GO WRONG?

Because the knee is so prone to injury, there is a tendency to think that all problems of the knee are caused by some traumatic event. The knee contains many kinds of tissues and is vulnerable not only to injuries, such as the tearing of a ligament, but also to arthritis and many other diseases. In addition, some injuries of the hip and lower leg appear initially to start in the knee as a result of a process called referred pain.

Knee problems can be the result of many different processes, some of them quite serious, so you should seek medical attention for any problem that does not clear up. In diagnosing a knee problem, a physician considers multiple possibilities even when the cause is relatively obvious. For example, an individual falls down and sustains a fracture. A physician, in inquiring about the injury, notes the fall was rather minor to produce such a major injury. He would be suspicious that the bone was abnormal to begin with and broke more easily than it should have. This approach suggests the possibility that some other disease process, such as a tumor, has seriously weakened the bone. One way that physicians solve problems in diagnoses is to categorize the possibilities by the origin or etiology. In looking at problems with the knee, the approach might be:

Congenital problems. The word "congenital" literally means you are born with the problem. Some infants are born with dislocated or excessively loose or lax knees. This condition can be the result of some very serious disease processes. Some people have

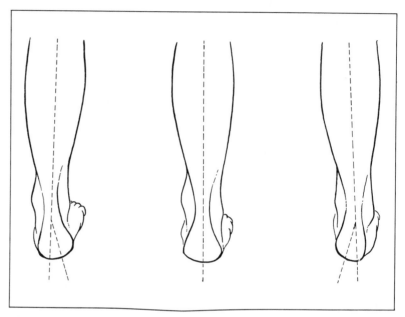

The alignment of the heel can influence the functioning of the knee. The heel on the left is angled outward (valgus). The center alignment is normal and the right alignment is abnormally inward (varus).

severe malalignment of the lower extremity which places abnormal stress on the joint. In addition, the cartilages may fail to form normally, which can lead to problems in later life.

Metabolic diseases. To function normally, the body depends on a delicate balance of many chemicals, including calcium, phosphorous and proteins, all necessary to form normal bones. Often, abnormally formed bone first becomes apparent when the bone fails. The knee, because of great stresses placed upon it, may be the weak link, and the first indication of a severe metabolic problem.

Inflammatory diseases. Arthritis and many similar conditions cause swelling, heat, pain and inflammation in the joint. These conditions may affect any joint in the body. However, the knee, perhaps because it is the largest and one of the most complex joints, seems particularly prone to certain types of arthritis. The various kinds of arthritis affecting the knee will be covered in a chapter on arthritis.

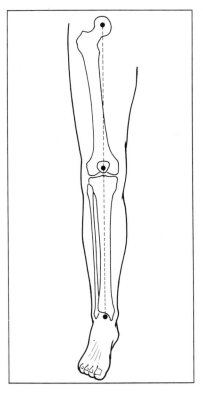

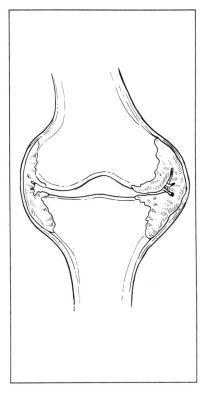

A well-aligned musculoskeletal system transmits weight from the hip to the knee and then to the ankle in a straight line.

In rheumatoid arthritis of the joints, the synovium or lining of the knee is responsible for a chemical reaction that leads to the destruction of cartilage.

Infection. An infection in the knee is a most serious condition demanding immediate attention. Infections can be caused by a bacterium, virus, fungus or even tuberculosis. Bacterial infections tend to produce rather rapid swelling and pain and, if not promptly controlled, may result in severe damage to the knee.

Tumors. Abnormal growths may occur anywhere in the body. The bones of the knee are among the fastest growing in the body and are affected frequently by very serious tumors. In many cases, these tumors are benign: The growth occurs only locally and, if excised, the patient will be cured. Some very serious cancers can also develop around the knee. The malignant bone tumor, osteosarcoma, frequently occurs there. A malignant tumor grows not only in the region where it starts, but the tumor cells may travel to other parts of the body and grow. Early identification and treatment of a tumor is the best hope for successful treatment.

Trauma. Knee injuries are now classified more specifically. In recent years, diagnosis of the specific site of injury has become much more precise. A physician generally categorizes trauma in terms of the tissue damaged—bone, ligament, tendon, muscle, capsule, nerves, vessels—as well as the energy and events responsible for the injury. (Specific injuries will be analyzed in a subsequent chapter.)

All of these conditions may appear similar to the person suffering from a knee problem. Some are simple and self-limiting while others are serious and potentially fatal. This uncertainty emphasizes the importance of seeking proper medical attention.

WHAT SHOULD I DO?

Gradual swelling. Swelling is the body's general response to an injured joint, particularly to such conditions as arthritis, damaged cartilage, infections or a bleeding disorder. The swollen joint may be caused by bleeding into the joint (hemarthrosis—heme for blood, arthrosis for joint), pus (pyarthrosis), or inflammation (effusion). Severe pain associated with swelling generally indicates the need for prompt medical attention. In some cases, swelling is not located in the knee joint itself, but in one of the bursae surrounding the knee, such as the pre-patellar bursa in front of the kneecap.

Sudden swelling. Swelling that comes on quickly, unassociated with any injury, particularly if there is fever, chills or merely a feeling of tiredness, requires immediate medical attention. This condition may indicate the presence of an infection or bleeding into the knee joint as in a disorder called hemophilia. The occurrence of swelling immediately after an injury indicates there may be serious damage to the ligaments of the knee. Medical consultation should be sought.

Giving out. Any knee that has been injured may give out. The causes may include weakness, a loose body, a fracture, a torn cartilage, a torn ligament or merely a response to pain. A knee which is unstable as a result of damaged ligaments may also give out long after the initial injury. While not an emergency, such a condition deserves careful medical attention.

Locked knee. In almost all cases, a knee locks because something mechanical is preventing it from functioning smoothly. Locking may result from a loose body (such as a piece of cartilage or bone), a dislocated kneecap or a torn meniscus which is stuck in the middle of the joint. These conditions require medical attention. Sometimes a previous injury may have weakened the structures of the knee, and even slight trauma may cause it to lock. On rare occasions, a sudden, painful injury may trigger an involuntary muscle spasm that holds the muscle so rigidly in one position that the knee appears to be locked.

Grinding. Grinding, referred to as crepitus by physicians, results when two rough surfaces rub against each other. The most common area for grinding is between the kneecap and the femur. Grinding may result when irregular, shaggy cartilage rolls over other irregular cartilage or even exposed bone, as in arthritis. The feeling may also be caused by loose bodies in the knee or by a torn cartilage positioned abnormally in the knee joint. If not painful, the condition may not be too serious.

Pain. A healthy knee does not hurt. Pain is an indication something is wrong. Location of the pain is the most important indicator of the cause of injury. In general, the more severe the pain, the sooner to seek medical attention.

Inability to walk on the knee. If a person can't walk on the knee after being injured, particularly following a high energy incident such as a football tackle, a skiing mishap or an automobile accident, medical attention should be sought promptly. If the inability to walk is associated with other problems such as paralysis, numbness or loss of feeling, a serious injury is likely.

Initial treatment of an injury. The diagnosis may not be known immediately following an injury, so certain basic principles should be followed for early treatment to decrease swelling and the likelihood of further injury. This treatment has been abbreviated as "RICE": **R**est, **I**ce, **C**ompression, **E**levation.

4

DIAGNOSING KNEE PROBLEMS

A **physician, in** diagnosing and treating a knee problem, begins by asking about the origin of the problem. He will want to know 1) how the problem began; 2) whether there are similar troubles, such as difficulty with the other knee or with other joints; and 3) whether there are any other current medical problems—perhaps a rash or a fever, sore throat or a myriad of other problems which your symptoms suggest.

When an injury is involved, he'll need to know the precise events: Just how did you fall? What happened? Did the knee swell up suddenly? Were you able to walk on the knee? Did you feel a pop? All questions are important in analyzing the cause of the problem. If you are a runner, a physician will ask about the type of running surface that seems to make the pain worse, whether going uphill or downhill has any effect, whether you've changed shoes lately, how far you can run before pain begins, what helps relieve the pain—all have a bearing in diagnosing knee problems.

If arthritis is involved, the physician will assess the degree of disability. How far can you walk before pain begins to bother you? Has the pain increased rapidly in recent days? What positions seem to be the worst? He will also want to know what effect previous treatment has had. Is the aspirin you are taking effective in relieving the pain? Does your knee pain wake you up at night?

EXAMINATION OF THE KNEE

After obtaining a complete history, learning how the problem began, the treatment to date, and the disability which has resulted, the physician will then perform a physical examination. The following are some of the highlights of that exam:

Inspection. Before even placing his hands on an extremity, the physician will scrutinize the leg to see if there's an obvious problem. In very severe injuries, an immediately visible deformity such as a fracture may be present. In other cases, the physician

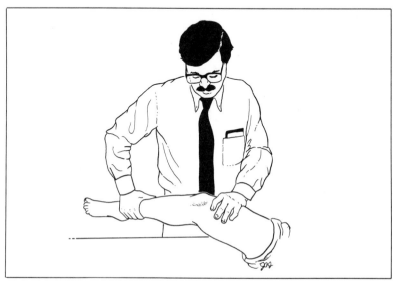

An orthopedic surgeon applies force to the side of the knee to test the medial collateral ligament.

will notice the knee is held in an abnormal position, as with a locked knee. Atrophy or muscle wasting may be evident. He will also look at the rest of the body to see if there are other signs of injury or a disease process affecting the whole body.

Motion of the knee. The physician will ask you to move your knee as far in all directions as you can. A variety of terms are used which may initially seem confusing, but they allow physicians to communicate with one another regarding the results of the examination. A knee which is completely straight is called *extended*. The act of straightening it is called *extension*. Bending the knee is referred to as *flexion*. Physicians refer to the motion of the knee as the *"range of motion."* The normal knee is able to bend from 0 degrees or full extension to approximately 140 degrees of flexion. When you are able to move the knee through this range of motion yourself, motion is referred to as *"active."* When you cannot, but another individual can move the knee through this motion, it is called *"passive."*

Fluid on the knee. Fluid on the knee indicates some injury. Physicians refer to the collection of fluid in a joint as an *effusion.* An

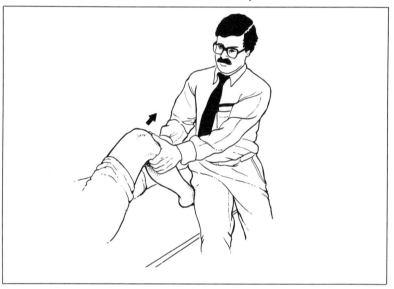

The anterior drawer exam. *The doctor pulls the knee forward to test the capsule and anterior cruciate ligament.*

effusion can occur as a result of virtually any insult to the joint. It is a very non-specific finding. Its presence merely indicates something is wrong; a sample of the fluid can be removed for analysis if necessary.

Stability of the knee. Many examinations have been devised to determine the integrity of ligaments of the knee. The physician applies a stress in one direction or another to see whether the ligament responsible for stabilizing the knee in that direction is competent and functioning. Pushing the knee to the outside or lateral side is referred to as a *valgus stress.* Pushing the knee to the inside or medial side is referred to as a *varus stress.* These maneuvers primarily reflect the competence of the respective collateral ligaments. The cruciate ligament and the capsule also help to stabilize the knee to sideward stress.

In some cases, a person will be in too much pain for a valid examination. The pain, plus the muscle spasm, may make testing of the ligament integrity impossible, and the joint may seem more stable than it really is. In such cases, an anesthetic may be required for the examination. This procedure is referred to as "exam under anesthesia."

Examination of the cruciate ligaments. The cruciate ligaments are responsible for preventing forward and backward motion of the tibia on the femur. The physician may perform an examination, called the Drawer examination, in which he pulls the knee either forward or backward to test whether the cruciates are present. In addition, the Lachman examination may be performed with the knee nearly straight and the physician pressing down above the kneecap and pulling up behind the tibia or shinbone. This procedure is also quite useful and actually more sensitive for determining the presence of an intact anterior cruciate ligament.

The unstable knee. A knee which is grossly unstable often shifts back and forth from the partially dislocated to the located position. Many different examinations have been devised to test stability—generally under the heading of the "pivot shift" examination. During this examination, the knee is twisted, and force is applied to one side of the knee, usually the outside. The knee is then straightened. When there is no functional capsule and cruciate ligament to restrain the knee, it partially dislocates with a palpable snap or slipping of one bone on the other. That's what happens when the knee gives out suddenly when someone with an unstable knee tries to make a cutting turn in basketball or runs sharply around a corner.

Tenderness. One of the most important aspects of a knee examination is the location of the pain. A physician will gently press on different areas of the knee, inquiring as to whether pain is located in each specific area. Pressing in the areas where cartilages are located may be the only objective indication that a meniscal tear has occurred. In addition, in many of the so-called *overuse*

syndromes of runners, the precise location of the pain is really
one of the most important factors in indicating the exact cause of
the knee problem.

Strength. Weakness of the muscles may be a contributing factor
to a knee problem. The strength of important muscle groups will
be tested.

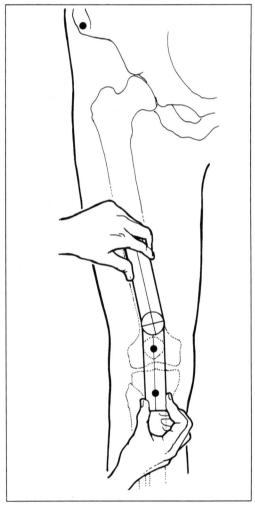

Q angle. *An important measurement for evaluation of the kneecap is the Q angle, which indicates the direction of pull of the quadriceps
muscle on the kneecap.*

The kneecap examination. The normal patella travels smoothly in the femoral groove. The physician will push the patella to test its stability and to determine if pain can be reproduced by direct pressure. He will also ask the patient to contract the quadriceps muscle and observe the dynamic path of the kneecap. A person with a previously dislocated patella will often wince with pain when the patella is pushed in the direction of dislocation—a maneuver referred to as a "positive apprehension sign." The physician will also determine the Q angle, a measurement of the alignment of the extremity. The Q angle gives an indication of the forces directed at the kneecap and the likelihood of a problem.

The foot examination. Disorders in the feet can be a cause of knee problems, particularly for runners. The alignment and mobility of the foot will be carefully evaluated to determine any effect on the knee. The wear pattern of the shoes is often an important clue to the diagnosis of abnormal foot mechanics. (See Runners' Injuries chapter.)

The hip examination. Disorders of the hip may appear to come from the knee. The hip will be moved through its arc of motion to determine any abnormality or if the pain is reproduced.

Gait. A normal gait requires a highly coordinated effort by the body. The walking pattern is an important part of the examination unless, of course, a recent injury has occurred. Sophisticated computerized gait analysis for special cases is now possible in some medical centers.

STUDIES FOR EVALUATING THE KNEE

Blood Studies

Certain blood components may give valuable information and clues to the cause of knee problems. For instance, when an infection is present in the knee, the body frequently responds with an outpouring of its protector cells—the white blood cells—resulting in an increased white blood cell count. Certain kinds of arthritis which affect the body as a whole, including the knee, have factors in the blood which indicate the presence of the disease. Rheumatoid factor and the anti-nuclear antibody are two. A frequently used test is called the erythrocytic sedimentation rate (abbreviated ESR): a rather imprecise indication that some significant disorder is taking place in the body. An individual with gout, which occurs when uric acid crystals form in a joint, very frequently has an elevated uric acid content in the blood. Over 1000 different tests can be performed on blood samples—some very complex and expensive. A physician carefully considers the potential diagnoses before requesting specific tests.

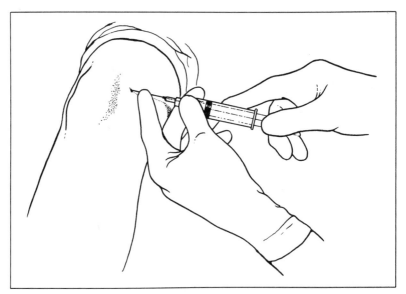

In some cases, removal and analysis of fluid in the knee joint may be necessary to diagnose a problem. This is known as an aspiration and is performed using sterile techniques.

Fluid on the Knee

When the knee is swollen, an analysis of the synovial fluid may prove invaluable. The type and number of blood cells is a fundamental indicator of the process responsible for the problem. If an infection is present, it is essential to know the exact cause. Is it a certain bacteria, fungus or perhaps tuberculosis? Initially, a special test called a gram stain is performed, which divides bacteria into two classes: gram positive—meaning that the bacteria pick up the stain, or gram negative—meaning they do not. The fluid is then placed in a special culture medium inside an incubator, and the bacteria, if present, will grow until they can be isolated and identified. The isolated bacteria are then tested using various antibiotics to see which would be most effective for eradicating the infection.

Uric acid crystals from an individual with gout can be seen in the fluid under a microscope. A special optical system called polarized light is used to analyze the crystals. Knowledge of the sugar and protein content as well as the stickiness of the fluid may aid in diagnosing particular knee problems. Blood found in the knee joint following a traumatic incident may indicate that a serious injury has occurred or, in some cases, that a blood clotting defect exists.

Nuclear Scans

The body constantly absorbs nutrients and supplies the cells with the particular substance they need to function normally. However, when some diseases or injuries are present, an abnormal amount of a particular chemical is concentrated in one area. A nuclear scan works because of this continuous absorption of nutrients. A small amount of radioactive material is introduced into the bloodstream attached to a substance used by the body. This substance is then concentrated where an abnormal process is present.

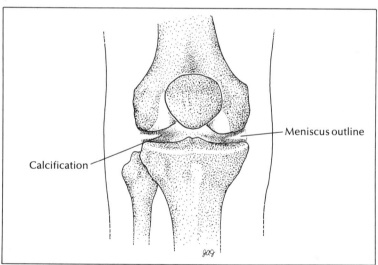

Calcification. Calcium crystals have precipitated in this joint and coated the cartilage.

For instance, the substance pyrophosphate is absorbed by the bone in a normal individual. In cases where there is an infection, a fracture or even a tumor, excessive amounts may be deposited in that region of the bone. By tagging this substance and then detecting it with a special scanner, physicians can discover abnormal regions of bone. Nuclear scans are particularly useful for early detection of a stress fracture, for instance. This injury is discussed in other sections. However, it should be noted that in many stress fracture cases, an X-ray of the bone appears normal for one to two weeks following the injury, but a nuclear bone scan shows the fracture only a few days after it occurs. In such a case, the cause of the pain can be established much sooner. Other chemicals can be tagged and used for detection of other abnormal processes.

When there is a question of infection, even white blood cells may have small amounts of radioactivity attached to them and can be followed to detect whether an infection is present and if so, where it is located. The amount of radioactivity contained in the nuclear material is minimal, and there is no current evidence that any harm occurs as a result of limited exposure to such a small amount of radioactivity.

X-Rays

X-rays (or roentgenograms) are essential for complete evaluation of the knee. An X-ray evaluation consists of an X-ray beam directed across the knee or any body part and onto special film. The dense bones block the passage of the rays, forming a shadow where bones or calcium are present. Fractures, bone diseases, tumors, arthritis, loose bodies and calcifications may all be seen on an X-ray. These films demonstrate abnormalities of the skeleton only. Injuries involving ligaments or cartilage cannot be seen on an X-ray.

There is appropriate concern by many individuals about exposure to X-rays. All responsible physicians take only those X-rays necessary to diagnose and treat a given problem. If you are pregnant or think you might be, you should, of course, notify your physician so X-rays will be avoided, if at all possible. Recently, there has been a considerable reduction in the amount of X-rays required to produce an image. In addition, the X-ray machines are able to direct the beam more precisely, minimizing the exposure of the rest of the body.

Ultrasound

Ultrasound is a technique which directs high frequency sound waves into the body to establish the presence of certain kinds of cysts or masses. One of the most common uses of ultrasound is in the diagnosis of obstetric problems, where physicians do not want to risk exposing the fetus to X-rays. There is no evidence to date that the limited use of ultrasound causes any birth abnormalities. However, only necessary use is recommended. In the knee, ultrasound can be particularly helpful for establishing the presence of a cyst.

Computerized Tomography

Quite recently, a new X-ray system has been developed which allows visualization of all structures of the body as if a cross-section were being created. X-rays are taken from many different angles and the information is fed into a computer to be analyzed. The images are then displayed on the screen in a fashion most useful to the radiologist. "CT" scanning allows precise visualization of tumors and other solid disorders around the knee.

Arthrograms

An arthrogram is a special X-ray of the joint taken after a dye has been injected into it. Cartilage is not seen in a regular X-ray picture, but in an arthrogram, dye injected into the knee coats the cartilage, making the knee joint cavity and the cartilaginous surface visible. Arthrograms are used primarily to evaluate tears of the meniscus (or cartilage). In addition, if there are any cysts, the dye may flow into them. For diagnosis of tears of the meniscus, this technique is 80 to 90 percent accurate.

Stress View X-Rays

In some cases of knee injury, the physician is uncertain whether the ligaments are intact and functional. When the knee is not too painful, the physician performs a stress view. This procedure involves taking an X-ray while a directional force is applied to the knee. In the illustration which follows, the knee is being pulled on, showing that the ligament which is supposed to hold the bones together is not functioning well, and it is possible to pull them apart. In children, there is often a question of whether an injury occurred at the growth plate or at a ligament. An X-ray stress examination will establish the diagnosis, and the extent of the injury can then be documented.

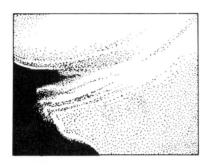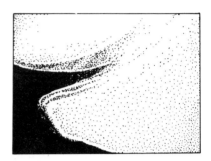

An arthrogram may show a torn cartilage. In a normal knee, the V-shaped wedge of cartilage is clearly outlined. When the cartilage is torn, the outline is irregular (left).

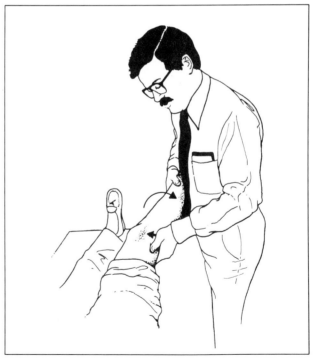

Applying stress to the knee while taking an X ray may reveal an injured ligament.

5

PROBLEMS OF THE BONE

Stress Fracture

The repeated leg pounding of running and marching may precipitate a stress fracture: a small area of micro-fracture where the bone is still in place but further trauma could result in sudden failure.

Stress fractures are found in only three animals—humans, race horses, and race dogs—in all cases resulting from overexertion. These fractures may occur anywhere in the lower extremities and are characterized by tenderness of the bone itself. They tend to occur more frequently in runners who overtrain, change running surface or shoes, or are in poor condition and stress their bodies beyond capacity. Stress fractures were originally labeled "march fractures" when they occurred with disturbing frequency among boot camp soldiers who were taken out on long marches without previous training.

One very disturbing product of the increasing involvement of children in organized athletics is the appearance of juvenile stress fractures. These fractures used to be extremely rare. In recent times, children have come under increasing pressure to excel in athletics. Clearly, this increased incidence of stress fractures is the result of overtaxing immature and vulnerable skeletons.

Treatment of stress fractures, to the dismay of devoted and inveterate runners, consists of rest and avoidance of stress on the involved bone. Stress fractures of the tibia rarely displace or require surgery, but continued running may significantly prolong healing. A person with a stress fracture is generally advised to participate in activities only as long as they don't cause pain. This approach generally requires stopping serious running for four to six weeks. Casts are generally not necessary, but if the pain persists, may be required to avert a complete fracture.

Intra-Articular Fracture

Fractures involving the knee joint may be very severe and, if not treated properly, may lead to instability and disabling arthritis. These injuries generally are caused by high-energy trauma such as automobile or motorcycle accidents or long falls. X-rays are necessary to identify the extent of the fracture. When the joint surface is fractured, it is important to determine the extent of the injury, as roughness or a ridge in the weight bearing portion of the joint may lead to uneven wearing and subsequent arthritis. When the fracture results in a significantly deformed joint, surgery is generally recommended to reconstruct the smooth joint surface.

Fractures in Children

In children, injuries frequently occur at the epiphyseal growth plate adjacent to the knee. The growth plate itself is actually weaker than the surrounding bone and ligaments; so when a severe injury occurs, the growth plate is more likely to be injured

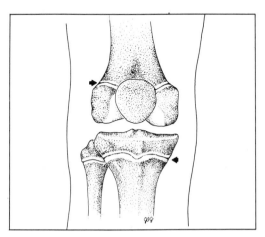

The top of the tibia and the bottom of the femur contain vitally important growth plates. These are areas of bone called epiphyses and are responsible for bone growth.

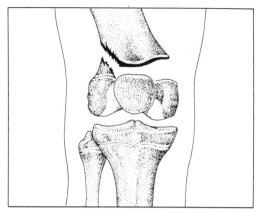

Growth plate fracture. *In children, the growth plate is weaker than the ligaments of the bone, and a blow to the knee may result in a fracture that travels through the growth plate.*

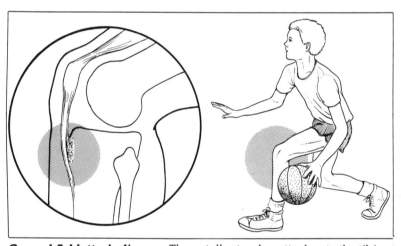

Osgood-Schlatter's disease. *The patellar tendon attaches to the tibia at a place where bone is growing. This area is frequently stressed in adolescents, leading to pain and swelling.*

than a ligament, as would occur in an adult. An injury to the growth plate may go completely through and not involve the joint, or a piece of the bone may be knocked off with the fracture extending into the joint. Careful treatment is necessary, particularly if the fracture is a severe one, because damage to the growth plate may result in a deformed or shortened leg. Treatment often requires surgery and placement of pins in the leg so that the bones are placed back precisely in their proper position. There is still the possibility of some permanent damage to the growth plate as a result of injury to the growth cells themselves.

Osgood-Schlatter's Disease

In this condition, the site where the patellar tendon attaches to the tibia becomes quite painful. There is a growth center of bone where the patellar tendon attaches, and during adolescence this area appears to be quite weak and prone to injury. The disease occurs primarily in teenagers who are actively growing. It is found in girls a couple of years sooner than boys because females reach skeletal maturity earlier. The pain is generally described as an ache and can be quite severe, particularly when a person tries to run or play sports. In most cases, resting from all painful activities will be adequate. A decrease in running distance, ice and anti-inflammatory agents may be helpful in mild cases. Sometimes normal activities are allowable, but the individual must not participate in physical education for a few months. When the pain is more severe, a splint may be necessary—worn either all the time or just at night. Surgery is rarely required.

Referred Pain

Pain that appears to come from the knee may actually originate in the hip. This symptom is particularly true in children and may indicate very serious hip disease. One such disease is called a slipped capital femoral epiphysis, caused by damage to the growth plate at the upper end of the femur. The nerve which produces pain in the hip area also supplies sensation to an area around the knee, and the signals are apparently confusing to the brain. This condition requires prompt attention by an orthopedic surgeon and is one reason why *a painful knee in a child is a condition which should be promptly evaluated by a family physician or an orthopedic surgeon.*

Another condition which is sometimes confusing is a "ruptured disc" or herniated nucleous pulposus. The nerves which supply sensation to the leg originate in the back. When a ruptured disc occurs, pressure may be applied to the nerves causing what is called radicular or radiating pain. This type of pain generally starts in the back and extends or radiates all the way down the leg. It can be quite severe and debilitating. Because it runs down the whole leg, there is sometimes confusion regarding its cause.

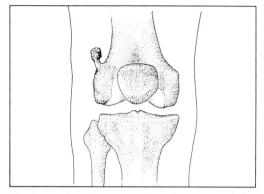

The knee is a frequent site of tumors of the bone. This one is an osteochondroma and should be removed if it causes problems.

Tumors

Growths or tumors in the area of the knee are rare but potentially quite serious. A tumor may be benign, which means that it grows locally, or may be malignant with a potential for uncontrolled growth and a capacity to travel to other parts of the body. A tumor may originate from bone as in osteosarcoma (a malignant tumor of bone) or from any other tissue in the knee. Unfortunately, there is nothing specific about the way a tumor feels, so any unusual persistent pain or any masses or growths should be evaluated. Sometimes, a tumor is first recognized when an injury occurs. For example, a very large cyst, involving most of the femur bone of the knee, might cause the bone to weaken and fracture. The individual was probably unaware of any problem in the bone. New techniques in surgery, radiation therapy and cancer chemotherapy now can offer a significantly better outlook for even very serious malignant tumors.

The Kneecap

One of the most common problems of the knee is pain around the kneecap (patella). This pain can be caused by many different conditions. The word "chondromalacia" has very frequently been used to refer to any pain in the area of the kneecap, but, technically, this term is not quite correct. "Chondromalacia" literally means softening of the kneecap and is a specific medical term referring to the condition on the cartilage on the underside of the kneecap.

Pain occurs when the patella rubs against the femur. This condition can result from trauma, such as a fall directly onto the knee, an unstable kneecap which rocks back and forth as it glides in the groove on the front of the femur (thighbone), or actual malalignment of the patellar mechanism and weakness of the quadriceps muscle. Patellar pain is found much more commonly in females than males, and is also one of the unfortunate consequences of running beyond one's capacity.

Determining the cause of patellar pain requires a careful evaluation. Females whose pelvises are broader tend to have muscles which pull the kneecap to the side, causing the kneecap to rub unevenly in the groove. Physicians refer to this condition as an increased Q angle, the angle formed by two intersecting lines, one drawn from the middle of the kneecap down to the tibial tubercle or place where the patellar tendon inserts on the tibia, and the second drawn from the middle of the kneecap up the shaft of the femur to intersect on a prominence on the pelvis. Clearly, if the pelvis is wider, the tendency would be for the kneecap to be pulled to the side. The force on the kneecap is increased by bending the knee and doing deep-knee bends. Adding weights during exercises to a knee that is angled may, in fact, make the condition worse rather than better.

Most individuals with patellar pain do not require surgery, although they do need a comprehensive treatment program of specific exercises, avoidance of certain activities and medication with anti-inflammatory drugs. In the vast majority of individuals, such a program will produce enough improvement to prevent surgery. Treatment of this pain may prove quite frustrating for many individuals; however, a cure is generally not rapid, and the pain is often recurrent. Fortunately, although many individuals suffer from patellar pain, some with chondromalacia, few will develop significant arthritis of the joint later in life.

The Partially Dislocating Kneecap

One of the consequences of malalignment or incongruity of the kneecap in the groove on the front of the femur is a tendency for the kneecap to partially dislocate or, as physicians refer to it, sublux. This condition is found more frequently in women than men and often requires surgical correction. However, an initial attempt is always made to treat the condition without surgery.

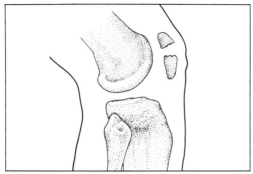

A severe blow to the patella may result in a fracture.

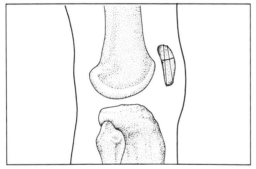

Repairing a fractured patella is important to prevent arthritis in the joint and to continue function of the quadriceps. Two pins have been placed to repair the fracture.

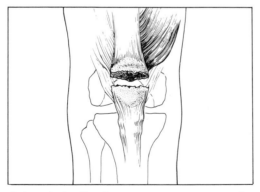

A break in the kneecap prevents muscles from straightening or extending the knee.

Special X-ray views are taken to demonstrate the abnormal position of the kneecap in the groove. Different measurements are then taken which show both the normal position of the kneecap as well as one tilted to the outside. This tilting makes the individual prone to partial dislocations and repeated episodes of pain. An additional condition, which predisposes one to a partially dislocating kneecap, is called femoral anteversion—a fancy term which means that the entire leg is turned in at the hip causing what is called "squinting kneecaps." These kneecaps point toward the middle and seem to face each other.

When kneecaps point inward, the muscles of the leg tend to pull the kneecaps outward, causing problems. This condition results from a failure of the body to derotate the legs into a normal condition following birth and tends to run in families. In childhood, these individuals frequently toe in. An individual with femoral anteversion can sit on his knees on the floor with the lower part of his legs out to the sides.

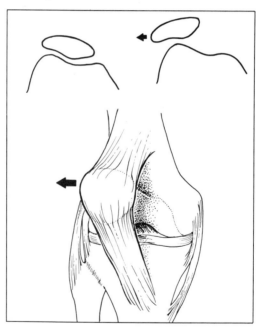

A sudden twisting motion accompanied by contraction of the quadriceps muscle may pull the kneecap to the side, causing a dislocation. Besides severe pain, a lump may appear on the side of the knee.

Treatment of the subluxing patella by most orthopedic surgeons proceeds sequentially starting with very simple and basic measures and progressing to surgery only if these fail. Specific surgery is discussed in the section on Surgery of the Knee.

The Fractured Kneecap

One consequence of falling on your knee can be to split the kneecap. The result is a total inability to straighten the leg. An X-ray will show the two fragments. In a younger individual, the fracture usually results in two major fragments. Older persons with weaker bones can have multiple fragments. The goal of treatment is to restore the bone to its normal position, perhaps with the placement of pins or wire to hold the fragments in place. In very severe cases, when the bone has been crushed beyond repair, actual removal of part or all of the kneecap may be required. Precise positioning of the fragments is important to prevent the development of arthritis in later life.

Dislocation of the Kneecap

Dislocation of the kneecap means it has slipped to the side of the knee. Quite frequently, an individual is able to relocate the kneecap before receiving medical attention. This condition is generally quite painful: One notices a lump out to the side of the knee, which is the kneecap.

Certain individuals with congenital knee deformities are more prone to dislocation. Surgery may be required to prevent multiple dislocations. However, the initial treatment is placement in a splint followed by a rigorous exercise program. The specific procedures are discussed in the section on knee surgery.

6

PROBLEMS OF THE LIGAMENTS

Severe injuries to the knee may result in tears of any or all of the ligaments. To return to normal, the torn structures must be identified and treated promptly. It is important to consult a physician immediately after the injury, because prompt treatment is far more effective. Examination may reveal the extent of the damage, but often an individual is in great pain and must be anesthetized to allow a complete examination. Evaluation of the contents of the joint with an arthroscope may reveal injuries not initially apparent. The term "sprain" applies to an injury limited to ligaments. Sprains can be graded according to the degree of damage:

First degree tear—tearing of a minimal number of fibers with localized tenderness but no instability.

Second degree tear—tearing of more ligament fibers with more loss of function but still no instability.

Third degree tear—complete disruption of ligament with instability of the joint.

Knee Stability

Ligaments are responsible for the stability of the knee. Physicians who treat knee problems refer to a knee as stable or unstable. A stable knee is capable of smooth, controlled motion. It does what you want it to do. An unstable knee moves in an abnormal way, is prone to giving out unpredictably, catching, swelling

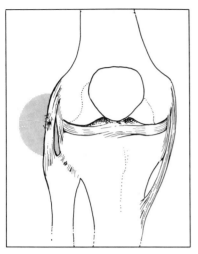

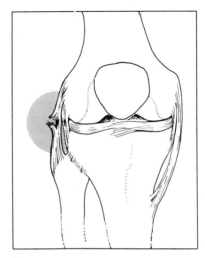

***Tear of lateral collateral liga-
ment.*** *When only a few fibers of a
ligament are disrupted, the tear is
referred to as a first-degree tear.*

***Partial tear of lateral collateral
ligament.*** *A ligament may be
damaged significantly but still
have some intact and functioning
fibers, which is referred to as a
partial or second-degree tear.*

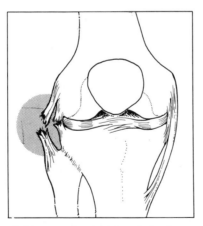

*A blow to the inside of the knee
may result in a complete tear of the
lateral collateral ligament on the
outside of the knee.*

and limiting activities. There are two basic types of stability:
1. Static stability (at rest)
2. Dynamic or functional stability

Static stability refers to a knee which has normal motion controlled by intact ligaments and capsule. This stability is determined by an examination of the knee at rest. Dynamic stability is the ability of the knee to respond to demands of the environment. This stability develops when the ligaments supplemented by the muscles surrounding the knee are able to balance and protect the knee from external forces.

A knee may be adequately stable for some activities, such as jogging, but not adequate for others such as basketball, where sudden, rapid movements are required. Stability is determined by the ability to function at the desired level of activity. Some individuals have significant static instability due to damaged ligaments but are able to participate in demanding sports because of the dynamic power of the muscles. There are significant variations from one person to another. Many people are born with lax (or loose) joints and are able to function quite well despite degrees of apparent instability which may be incapacitating to others. An individual sometimes can learn to adapt to the known instability of a joint by changing his jumping pattern or avoiding twisting motions on the unstable side.

There are many different types of instability. Currently, physicians use a system which describes the type of instability by the direction in which the tibia moves abnormally in relation to the femur. There are two basic classes of unstable knees. In the straight type, the knee is unrestrained in one plane: It moves too far forward or backward, or moves too much to the inside or outside. In the rotatory type, the knee is capable of uncontrolled rotation of one bone upon the other with the posterior cruciate ligament serving as the center of rotation.

The two most common types of rotatory instability are anterolateral and anteromedial. In anterolateral instability, the outside of the knee joint (or lateral tibial plateau) rotates forward in relation to the femur as a result of damage to the anterior cruciate ligament, the capsule, and the arcuate ligament complex. In anteromedial instability, just the opposite happens. The inside of the knee rotates outward in relation to the femur as a result of damage to the anterior cruciate ligament, medial collateral ligament and posterior oblique ligament.

These descriptions are all very confusing. Do not be too disheartened, though, as the determination of instability is a highly complex process even for experienced orthopedic surgeons. To further complicate matters, it is possible to have many combinations of these instabilities from more severe injuries. Identification of the precise instability is extremely important, as surgery to correct the damage must be directed at the proper structures.

KNEE INSTABILITY

Type	Primary Injury	Secondary Injury
Medial	medial collateral	anterior cruciate posterior oblique
Lateral	lateral collateral	anterior cruciate arcuate complex
Posterior	posterior cruciate	capsule
Anterior	anterior cruciate	capsule
Antero- lateral	anterior cruciate	arcuate complex capsule
Antero- medial	anterior cruciate	medial collateral posterior oblique

The Torn Medial Collateral Ligament

The medial collateral ligament is responsible for maintaining the inside of the knee joint in proper position. A sideways stress to the joint may result in damage to this ligament. This injury can occur in an automobile accident where a bumper strikes the knee or from a direct blow to the knee in football. Falls also can tear the medial collateral ligament, but they tend to be partial.

When the medial collateral ligament is completely torn and no other injury is present, most orthopedic surgeons now recommend a cast followed by controlled motion in a cast brace—a hinged cast which allows motion of the joint but which protects the ligament. Partial tears of the ligament are treated with protected motion, crutches and a gradual return to stressful activities. A cast brace may be recommended for some individuals. In cases where the tear is associated with more significant injuries, surgery may be recommended. In some cases, pain is so severe that the degree of damage cannot be determined just from the

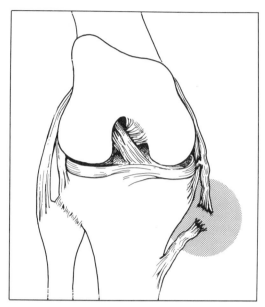

*A blow to the outside of the knee may cause
the medial collateral ligament to tear.*

examination. An anesthetic must then be given and the knee examined with the individual asleep.

The Torn Lateral Collateral Ligament

The lateral collateral ligament is responsible for maintaining the outside of the knee in the proper position. A blow to the inside of the knee is generally responsible for causing a tear of the lateral collateral ligament. The knee tends to open up or go to the outside whenever weight is applied. In general, tears of the lateral collateral ligament are also associated with tears of the capsule in the back of the knee and in the area called the arcuate ligament, a Y-shaped collection of stabilizing structures in the back of the knee. When the lateral collateral ligament has been completely torn, surgical repair is generally recommended.

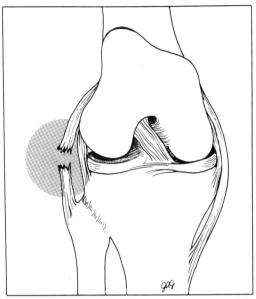

*The lateral collateral ligament, responsible
for restraining the outside of the knee, may be
torn by a blow to the inside of the knee.*

The Terrible Triad

One fairly common football injury is actually a combination of injuries known by orthopedic surgeons as the "terrible triad"—tears of the medial collateral ligament, the medial meniscus, and the anterior cruciate ligament. This injury is extremely severe, and, in almost all cases, surgery is recommended.

Dashboard Knee

In an automobile accident, the knee may be driven into the dashboard when the car suddenly stops. The use of seatbelts has drastically reduced these injuries, but they still occur. Multiple injuries are possible, too. One of the most common is damage to the posterior cruciate ligament, the structure responsible for keeping the tibia from moving backward on the femur. In more

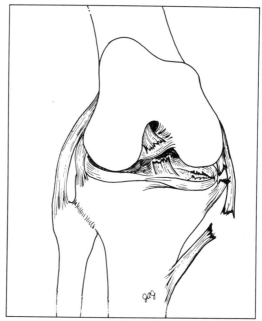

A severe knee injury called "the terrible triad" consists of a torn medial collateral ligament, medial meniscus and anterior cruciate ligament.

severe cases, a complete dislocation of the knee, often with rupture of the popliteal artery—the main artery of the leg—may result. This injury requires a very careful, prompt evaluation.

The Torn Anterior Cruciate Ligament

The anterior cruciate ligament is one of the most important ligaments in the knee. It is responsible for 85 percent of the restraining force that keeps the knee from being pulled forward. It also keeps the knee from rotating abnormally and from being pulled to the outside. The anterior cruciate ligament may be torn in a fairly isolated injury (along with damage to the capsule), or it may be part of a more massive injury, involving the collateral ligaments and the menisci. A typical isolated tear of the anterior cruciate ligament may occur in a non-contact incident as when a running back in football plants his foot and then decelerates while twisting the knee. He may feel a pop and have immediate and severe pain. This reaction may be followed by an inability to walk

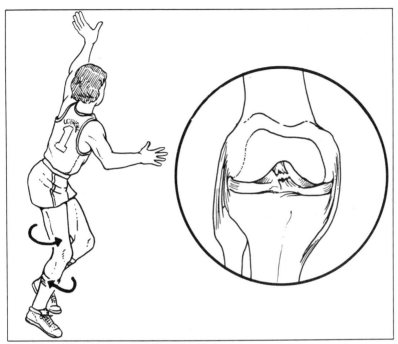

A sudden twisting movement in which the leg is planted and the body twisted forcefully may result in a torn anterior cruciate ligament.

on the knee and, within two hours, the development of severe swelling. In other cases, where a severe blow is delivered to the knee, a collateral ligament along the side of the knee, as well as the cruciate ligament, may be torn.

Dramatic advances have been made in the diagnosis and treatment of tears of the anterior cruciate ligament. Many concepts held dear by many surgeons a few years ago have been found to be incorrect. We now know that an individual who sustains a significant knee injury with immediate swelling from bleeding, has approximately a 60 to 70 percent chance of having a torn anterior cruciate ligament. This tear is far more frequent than was previously believed. Because the knee is often so painful, diagnosis of an anterior cruciate ligament tear may be difficult. For some individuals, the diagnosis is quite clear, and the performance of stress examinations by the physician (the Drawer examination and the Lachman examination) clearly demonstrate a torn ligament. For others, an anesthetic may be necessary to evaluate the stability of the ligaments. Arthroscopy may be needed to determine additional damage to the knee.

What Happens if the Ligament Is Torn?

The anterior cruciate ligament is important for optimal functioning of the knee. Even so, an individual can have a torn ligament and experience little or no functional disability. For many individuals whose activities are limited, repair of a torn anterior cruciate ligament is not necessary. Casting or bracing, and a vigorous exercise program following the injury may enable them to pursue all of their normal activities. For some, normal activities may cause no problems, but there may be significant limitations in vigorous athletics which require jumping, cutting, and sharp turns, such as football, racquetball or basketball. Jogging on level ground is often no problem. These individuals must then decide whether such activities are important enough to warrant undergoing a fairly major operation and a very prolonged rehabilitation program following the initial injury.

For other patients, the anterior cruciate ligament tear and the associated instability may prove disabling. This disability may range from the knee catching and giving out with virtually every step, to occasional swelling and pain if any sort of athletics is attempted. These individuals, if in good health and if they want to

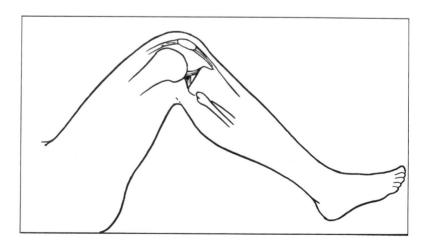

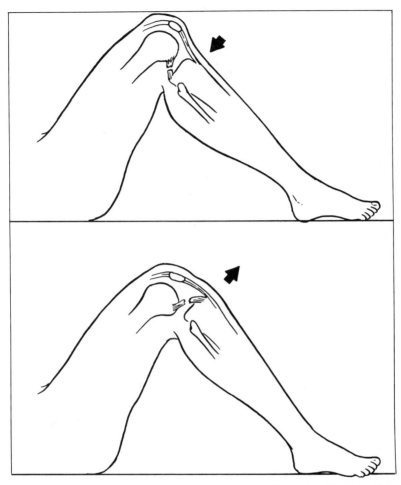

The cruciate ligaments. *Opposite page: Normal knee in which the tibia sits in its proper place in respect to the femur. Top: Torn posterior cruciate ligament. Bottom: Torn anterior cruciate ligament.*

continue to maintain a high activity level, may be candidates for surgery. There is some evidence that chronic or long-term instability of the knee as a result of a torn anterior cruciate ligament may lead to degenerative arthritis in later life. Such individuals are also more prone to tears of their menisci (cartilages).

Bracing may also be useful in stabilizing the knee. A special rotation brace is required. An Ace wrap or a simple hinge brace will not furnish adequate stability for the individual to pursue vigorous activities. A brace is only part of treatment, however, and no substitute for proper rehabilitation.

As you can see, treatment of a torn anterior cruciate ligament tear is highly complex. The term "anterior cruciate deficient knee" is now used by some to describe a knee with a torn ligament; but the more important description is the resulting degree and type of instability. A physician must consider not only the physical injury, but also the general health of the individual, his other problems and his desires for future activity. Some individuals may demand that everything medically possible be done to restore an injured knee to normalcy. Others want an operation only if absolutely necessary. Physicians recognize that any surgery must be followed by a lengthy and vigorous exercise program that is highly dependent upon the commitment and determination of the individual. No surgery is recommended unless a person is highly motivated to rehabilitate his knee. The goal of surgery is to restore stability, not just replace the anterior cruciate ligament. There are many different surgical procedures and rehabilitation programs recommended, reflecting the fact that new knowledge is rapidly being generated. The long-term results of many of these procedures are not known. Therefore, physicians must make their decisions based on the best available information, realizing that it is incomplete. That's why you may hear divergent opinions concerning treatment of tears of the anterior cruciate ligament. (This topic is discussed in more detail in the knee surgery chapter.)

7

PROBLEMS OF THE JOINT AND CARTILAGE

Many problems can afflict the knee joint and cartilage. Following are descriptions of some of the major problems, including osteochondritis dissecans, Baker's cyst, torn meniscus, plica, synovitis, infection and loose body.

Osteochondritis Dissecans

Occasionally, a piece of bone and cartilage may separate from the surface of the knee joint. A child with this condition typically complains of a vague soreness, swelling and pain during activities requiring repetitive flexion such as running, bicycling and deep knee bends. In 30 percent of these cases, both knees are affected. The separation is found on the inside of the medial femoral condyle in 75 percent of these cases.

The piece may remain in place and cause pain, or may break off and become a loose body in the knee. Problems may be caused by the joint surface, now defective, and from the effect of a free piece of bone and cartilage in the joint. If recognized early in young children, the condition will often heal itself if stress is removed from the knee. Frequently, the only treatment necessary is to curtail vigorous athletics. In older adolescents, surgery may be required to treat the loose fragment: drilling holes into the bones at the site of the defect in the cartilage to encourage the formation of a fibrous type of cartilage. If the bony fragment has remained in place, it can often be firmly secured with pins or a screw.

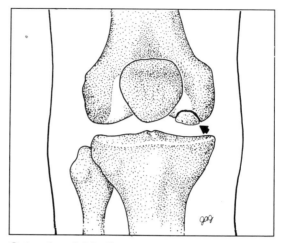

Osteochondritis dissecans. *A piece of bone and cartilage may loosen from its attachment to the femur and cause a lesion. These lesions generally heal if properly treated.*

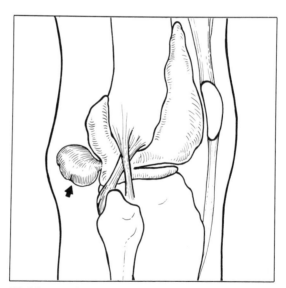

Fluid sometimes collects in a small cyst—called a Baker's cyst—behind the knee. Sometimes the cyst will grow to enormous size.

Baker's Cyst

A pocket of fluid may collect outside of the joint. When fluid collects behind the knee, it is commonly known as a Baker's cyst. Patients with rheumatoid arthritis are quite prone to develop this cyst. It is generally not painful but may indicate some other problem which affects the mechanics of the knee. Often, the knee generates a large amount of fluid which is pushed into the cyst, causing it to become so large that it fills up the entire back of the leg. In these cases, the cyst may appear to be a blood clot. Sophisticated testing, such as a venogram, may be necessary to distinguish the cyst from the more serious blood clot. In many cases, treatment of the problem inside the knee with arthroscopy may result in elimination of the Baker's cyst. Surgical removal is rare and only necessary when the cyst does not respond to simpler measures.

INJURIES OF THE CARTILAGE

Torn Meniscus

A common injury among young, active persons is a tear of the meniscal cartilage. However, since the advent of arthroscopy, physicians are now seeing an increasing frequency of tears in older individuals. A torn meniscus may cause problems such as a suddenly locked knee, a dull ache with activity, swelling, clicking, snapping or a feeling of catching. Sometimes the clicking may even be audible. Pain is generally localized along the joint line of the involved cartilage. In many cases, the tear is not the result of a single massive injury but rather is caused by chronic stress on a weakened cartilage. The knee may give out or seriously lock when the torn cartilage is pushed into the middle of the knee joint. Activities such as squatting may cause severe discomfort. Tears of the medial meniscus occur five times more commonly than tears of the lateral meniscus and are more common in males.

In the past, treatment consisted of excision of the entire cartilage (total meniscectomy, a procedure requiring a surgical incision and a prolonged rehabilitation). Arthroscopy and arthroscopic surgery have changed this treatment. Now, in most cases, when a tear occurs, only the involved portion of the meniscus is removed through arthroscopic surgery (see arthroscopy chapter).

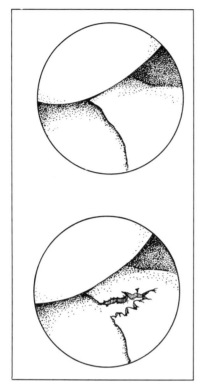

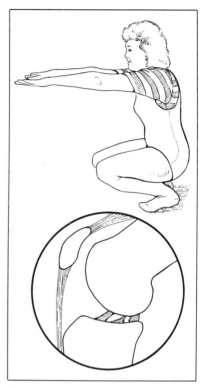

Torn cartilage. *The top illustration shows a view through an arthroscope of a normal cartilage; the bottom illustration shows a jagged tear in the cartilage.*

Torn meniscus. *Doing a deepknee bend can lead to a torn cartilage in a susceptible person. When this happens the meniscus is crushed between the femur and tibia.*

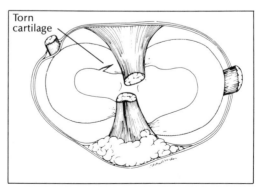

Torn
cartilage

A small tear in the meniscal cartilage can cause major problems.

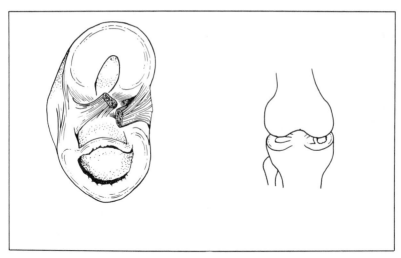

A meniscus may be torn so badly that part of it is pushed into the middle of the knee.

In certain cases, the meniscus can actually be sewn back together. New techniques are constantly being developed for this procedure, and time will tell whether the repairs will prove lasting. In the past, studies have shown that individuals who underwent total removal of the meniscus were more likely to develop arthritis on the side involved. It is hoped that partial removal of a torn meniscus (leaving the normal cartilage in place) or sewing a torn meniscus back together will be less likely to lead to arthritic changes in the joint.

Plica

A plica is a band of tissue, generally along the medial side of the knee, which may cause pain as it rubs against the side of the bone. The band is present in many individuals but probably causes pain in only a few. There may be snapping or an aching sensation brought on by running or stair climbing. Many individuals respond to a relatively simple therapy such as an exercise program, modified activities, and treatment with anti-inflammatory medications and ice. When these measures fail and the symptoms are severe, surgery may be necessary to remove the band of tissue. A diagnosis can be made by arthroscopy, and surgery may usually be performed arthroscopically.

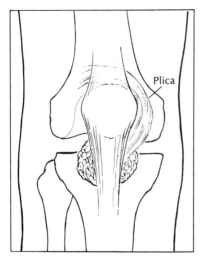

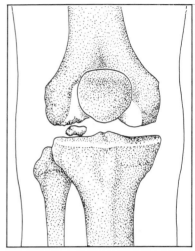

Plica. *An abnormal band of tissue present in the knee may cause pain in some individuals. Most of the time this band is located on the medial side of the knee.*

A piece of bone or cartilage may break off the knee and float freely. A loose body that becomes stuck between the femur and tibia is one cause of a locked knee.

Synovitis

When the synovium of the knee is stimulated, it pours out a large amount of fluid and causes swelling: commonly called "water on the knee." This "effusion," as it is called by physicians, may be caused by many different diseases or injuries and is the body's attempt to protect the knee from further injury. The stimulus might be a mechanical problem or even an early form of arthritis. If you have an effusion, medical attention should be sought.

Infection

An infection of the knee is very serious; it requires immediate examination by a physician. An infection can be identified by a sudden swelling of the knee with redness, severe pain and often an inability to straighten the knee. Fever, chills and a feeling of fatigue may occur. Infection somewhere else in the body often precedes the development of infection in the knee. Bacteria, fungi, viruses and even tuberculosis can infect the knee. Because treatments are different, dependent on the type of infection involved, it is crucial to identify the organism.

When an infection is suspected, fluid is extracted from the knee and sent for special stains and cultures. The appropriate treatment can then be prescribed. An infection in the knee produces chemical substances which can destroy the cartilage and cause arthritis. Removal of this fluid with a needle is sometimes required. If this treatment is not adequate, drainage through an operation may be necessary. The goal is to protect the cartilage from damage by the chemicals produced by the bacteria. Treatment requires that the patient be hospitalized and receive intravenous antibiotic medications. In teenagers and young adults, the most common cause of an infected knee is gonorrhea. The bacteria, initially introduced into the body by sexual contact, travel through the bloodstream and may ultimately infect any joint, frequently the knee. The infection is often preceded by a vague aching in the wrist and pain which seems to travel from one joint to another. If recognized early and treated properly, most individuals with an infection of the knee joint recover completely.

Loose Body

A piece of cartilage or bone may sometimes dislodge and float loosely inside the knee joint. It may cause the knee to grind or it may become lodged between the femur and tibia and cause the knee to lock. In many cases, a small loose body may be removed by arthroscopy. In other cases, more major open traditional surgery may be required.

8

PROBLEMS OF THE SOFT TISSUES

The tissues around the knee are prone to injury and inflammation, often precipitated by athletics. Running, in particular, places repetitive strain on the knee.

Tendinitis

A tendon connects muscle to bone but is not part of a joint. Friction along the tendon, whether between the tendon and its surrounding sheath or between the tendon and another structure, is called tendinitis. Inflammation may also occur when there has been failure of some of the tendon fibers (a partial tear).

Rest, supplemented with anti-inflammatory medication and ice, is the primary therapy for tendinitis. Injection with corticosteroids may be helpful in some cases, but this treatment increases the possibility of a tendon rupture. (See cortisone injection section.)

Patellar Tendinitis (Jumper's Knee)

Pain around the patellar tendon is often called "jumper's knee" because it frequently occurs in high jumping, kicking and running. The pain generally follows explosive, repetitive activities and is often associated with poor training habits. Swelling along the tendon may be present, and if the tendinitis is long-standing, fibrous tissue may develop. Treatment is directed at relief of the precipitating factors, often requiring rest and modification of training. Ice and anti-inflammatory medication are the initial treatments. Steroids can be injected into the tendon area, but this treatment is dangerous and may result in a ruptured tendon. When pain treatments fail, surgical removal of inflamed scar tissue may be necessary for relief.

Fibrositis

Fibrositis is a rather confusing condition. Muscular pain for which no specific explanation can be found is classified under this illness. A number of terms have been used to describe fibrositis, including musculoskeletal pain syndrome, muscular rheumatism, fibromyalgia, myofasciitis, and non-articular rheumatism. The condition is known for pain that occurs at sites on the body often called trigger points. These areas are tender and seem to be places where muscle or the covering over muscle, called fascia, is either stressed or irritated. Once the pain begins, a vicious cycle can occur: The muscles react to protect the painful area, causing spasm and more pain.

Fibrositis occurs more in women than men and also is found in persons who are tense, anxious, or having emotional difficulty with depression, anger or frustration. Many diagnostic studies are performed, primarily to eliminate the possibility of other serious conditions. All X-ray studies and blood tests are normal. Treatment can be extremely difficult, and often including medication for pain. Physical therapy and ultrasound can help greatly. When a specific emotional stress is involved, psychotherapy may help. When the condition is made worse by an occupational requirement, changing jobs may be necessary. Surgery is never advised but injections of pain medications and steroids may dramatically help to interrupt the pain from a trigger point.

Cramps

Cramps are caused by the involuntary contraction of a muscle. This condition frequently occurs at night and is found especially in swimmers, people who exercise without adequate warmup, and people with disorders of metabolism involving sodium, the thyroid gland and the kidney. In rare cases, cramps may be a symptom of very serious neurologic problems or of a fundamental disorder of muscle metabolism. Whatever the cause, the muscle contracts even though it is in a resting, shortened position. Quite often, a "knot" in the muscle can be felt.

While there is much yet to learn, we do know cramps are

caused by excessive discharge of the motor nerves. Often, the condition can be successfully treated by stretching and massage; medication is sometimes necessary to stabilize nerve membranes and prevent them from contracting the muscle. Quinine is the classically used medication and is often successful. Other drugs such as Tegretol and Dilantan are also helpful to some. For cramps that seem to be brought on by exercise, a regular program of stretching prior to a workout may help.

Contusion

A contusion is an injury to the muscles and tissues caused by a blow from a blunt object. The quadriceps muscle is particularly prone to the contusion type of injury in contact sports. Contusions are often quite painful , and swelling may occur from bleeding into the muscle. Initial treatment attempts to relieve the pain and control bleeding, usually including the application of ice and rest. Once the pain has subsided, progressive exercises and heat are recommended.

Bruise

A bruise is an injury sustained from a blunt object which does not break the skin. Rupture of small blood vessels leads to swelling and discoloration of the skin. Application of ice and pressure to control bleeding are the initial recommended treatments.

Hematoma

Hematoma refers to a collection of blood in the tissues. When the quantity is excessive, drainage may be recommended. For minor injuries, the body's protective mechanism will gradually resorb the fluid.

Muscle Strain

A muscle strain occurs when excessive tension has stretched a muscle beyond its limit. Weak and overused muscles are more prone to injury. In very sudden injuries, the muscle may be torn from the bone or a fragment of bone may be pulled off with the muscle, an injury referred to as an avulsion fracture. This bony fragment is visible on an X-ray.

The hamstrings seem particularly prone to stretching injuries which are particularly painful. Treatment requires rest and initial application of ice. Once the early pain has subsided, a program of progressive stretching should be started, followed by resistive exercises and finally a gradual return to athletics. Far too many individuals fall victim to recurrent injuries while trying to return too rapidly to activities with an improper training program.

Bursitis

Whenever two structures in the body slide past one another, a bursa, or pouch, is formed between them. Bursitis is the inflammation of the bursa from friction or irritation. There are usually 14 different bursae in the knee. The pes anserinus and popliteus bursae often become irritated in long-distance runners. The prepatellar bursa, located just in front of the kneecap, may become painful and swollen from direct pressure on the knee. This condition is common among persons who spend considerable time kneeling and has been called "housemaid's knee." It is particularly common among carpet layers.

Treatment of bursitis initially demands resting the extremity to prevent repeated irritation. Anti-inflammatory medications and ice packs may be prescribed. Injections of corticosteroid into the region of irritation may also be recommended. For runners who develop a bursitis, pre-treatment before running with an anti-inflammatory medication, such as aspirin, and icing of the area immediately following the run may prove helpful.

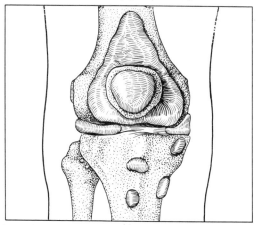

The knee is surrounded by many bursae or small sacs at locations where friction occurs over the joint.

9

RUNNERS' INJURIES OF THE KNEE

The enthusiasm of runners is often greater than the ability of the knee to withstand the repeated stress required of the sport. At a running cadence of 200 steps/min for 5 hours/week (40 miles), each limb will undergo the following number of cycles: 100/minute, 6000/hour, 30,000/week, 1,560,000/ year. (Winter,D. A., *Biomechanical Analysis of the Kinetics of Jogging*, Dept. of Kinesiology, University of Waterloo, Waterloo, Ontario, 1984.) Two out of every three joggers are afflicted by some injury each year,and 25 to 35 percent of these injuries involve the knee. The majority of all running problems are caused by errors in training—for both the marathon runner and the weekend jogger.The following factors are likely to lead to orthopedic problems and injuries:

- Dramatic change in the pattern of running
- A change in the running surface or contour
- New shoes
- Inadequate warmup
- Increased mileage
- Malalignment of the lower extremity
- Previous joint abnormality
- Muscular weakness and imbalance

Many problems unique to the runner are caused by overuse. Mechanically, jogging exerts a repetitious, high-impact force on the knee joint that may approach three to four times the body's weight. All joints in the lower extremity are affected, but the knee is the most susceptible to injury.

Kneecap Problems

Problems of the patella are particularly common in runners. Patellar pain is the most prevalent condition limiting the distance individuals are able to run. Most kneecap problems are the result of overuse injuries. Many terms, including lateral compression syndrome and patello-femoral stress syndrome, have been used to describe pain in this area. As discussed in the kneecap section (Chapter 5), malalignment of the lower extremity from femoral anteversion or knock-knees may intensify problems of the patella. Running brings out malalignment problems which might not have surfaced if constant repetitive force had not been placed across the joint. Deformities of the foot—in particular, the so-called "pronated foot"—may also place undue stress across the patello-femoral joint.

Iliotibial Band Syndrome

One particularly important training consideration is the contour of the running surface. Running on the side of a hill is certain to place imbalanced force across the knee joint due to the rotation of the leg, the twisting angulation of the foot, and the pull of the ligaments. The repeated motion may provoke an iliotibial syndrome. The iliotibial band is a strong bundle of fibers which travels along the lateral or outside of the femur and connects to the upper portion of the tibia. Irritation of this area occurs almost exclusively in marathon runners, particularly if they're running

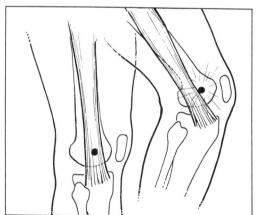

Iliotibial band syndrome. *In some people, the iliotibial band, which helps stabilize the knee, may become painful when it rubs over the outside of the femur.*

on hills or uneven surfaces. Treatment attempts to relieve irritation through modification of running shoes, change of terrain, stretching of the iliotibial tract before running, ice, cortisone injections and anti-inflammatory medication. Surgery is rarely needed.

Popliteus Tendinitis

A small muscle on the back of the knee, the popliteus, develops tendinitis almost exclusively from frequent downhill running. Successful treatment requires a change of running pattern and, like other types of tendinitis, ice, anti-inflammatory medications and rest.

Pes Anserinus Bursitis

The pes anserinus bursa is a commonly inflamed area in runners. The muscles which promote internal rotation of the tibia attach to the bone by means of the pes anserinus tendon. Runners who jog on tracks with sharply banked sides are particularly vulnerable to problems, presumably because of the sudden, forceful, rotatory movements required to negotiate the turns. Treatment consists of changing terrain, decreasing mileage, and rest, if the bursitis is particularly painful. Orthotics may help some individuals. Ice, anti-inflammatory medications and, on occasion, a corticosteroid injection may lead to relief.

The Pronated Foot

Runners have long known that injuries and deformities of the foot may cause serious knee problems. Physicians have recently recognized the great effect pronation of the foot can have on the knee. Pronation is a rather complex concept. Basically, it implies a rotation of the foot inward so that more weight is carried on the inside of the foot. In running, the foot normally pronates, which provides some springiness to the foot and helps protect joints of the lower extremity from excessive force. However, in some individuals, due either to weakness or some inborn predisposition, this pronation is excessive. The rotation is transmitted from the forefoot, or front of the foot, to the hindfoot, or the heel, and then up the leg where internal rotation or a turning in of the tibia occurs. When examining a runner who is having problems, physicians look at the heel's position. Normally, the heel is vertical. In a seriously pronated foot, the heel is in valgus or pointed outward. The result is a rotation of the tibia and a tendency for the mechanics of the knee to be disturbed. Patellar problems are quite common in individuals with a pronated foot.

Treatment of the pronated foot requires placement of inserts in the shoe. Simple, off-the-shelf inserts are quite adequate for some runners. For others, custom inserts may be necessary to stabilize the foot and prevent rotation from being transmitted up the leg. Some running shoes currently have stabilizers on the heel to help prevent some of this rotation.

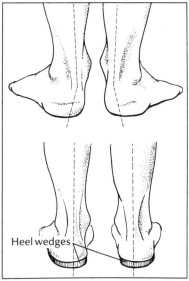

The feet have a profound effect on the function of the knee. Top illustration: The heels are angled outward (valgus), a condition that may lead to knee problems. Heel wedges may bring the heel into alignment.

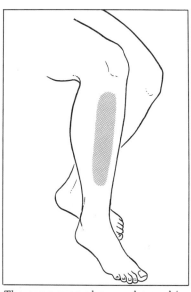

The gray area shows where shinsplints commonly occurs. This injury is the scourge of beginning runners.

Shinsplints

The term "shinsplints" is a general term used to describe pain occurring along the shinbone (tibia). There are numerous causes of this pain, and the diagnosis may prove quite difficult. The pain may be caused by muscle tears, detachment of the muscle from the bone after multiple tears in the ligaments, a stress fracture, a compartment syndrome or a pronated foot. Different terms, such as periostitis, have also been used to indicate that the periostium, the tissue which surrounds the bone, has been damaged. This damage is generally the consequence of overpull by an attached ligament.

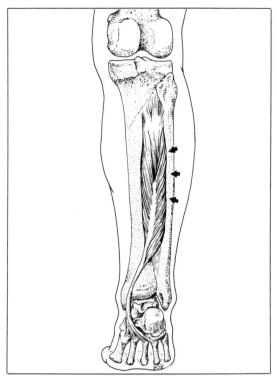

*One cause of shinsplints is excessive force on the
bone where the posterior tibial tendon attaches.
This may be caused by a foot angulated improp-
erly so that it transmits excessive force to the posterior tibial tendon and muscle.*

The posterior tibial muscle is a powerful muscle attached to the
back surface of the tibia. It travels down across the ankle and an-
chors on the inside of the foot. Chronic overpull of this muscle
where it attaches to the bone is sometimes responsible for causing pain. A person with a pronated foot who rotates the foot outward places an extra pull on the muscle, and this action may be
one of the causes of shinsplints. A correction of the pronated foot
will, in many cases, resolve this problem. Because so many different conditions may cause shinsplints, pain which persists deserves a careful and complete evaluation.

Compartment Syndrome

A compartment syndrome is a rare complication of running,
strenuous activity or injury involving the lower extremity. The
problem has been recognized for many years. The most serious
form was described as "march gangrene" when found in military

recruits who were required to go on long, forced marches. The muscles of the leg are surrounded by a rather inflexible covering of tissue called fascia which has a limited ability to expand. There are four separate compartments in the leg, each having its own blood and nerve supply to the muscles in the compartment. Normally, there is plenty of room for the muscles to expand and contract. Following overuse or a severe injury, however, the muscles and tissues may swell so much that the blood vessels are compressed and the blood supply to the limbs is diminished or cut off. Poorly conditioned individuals are particularly likely to develop this syndrome.

In a compartment syndrome, the pain and swelling occur following a strenuous activity and are quite severe. Often, there is tingling in some of the toes, and movement is extremely painful. A compartment syndrome may be chronic and self-limiting, meaning that it comes and goes with strenuous activity, or it may be acute and cause irreversible damage if emergency surgery is not performed to restore the blood flow. Any time you have a pain which seems largely out of proportion to what you might expect and does not respond to simple analgesics, seek prompt medical attention. Irreversible damage may occur if the problem is left untreated. Surgical treatment consists of releasing the pressure on the muscle by opening up the compartment, a procedure called a fasciotomy.

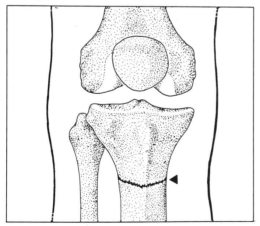

Stress fracture. *A repetitive activity such as jogging may cause a stress fracture. The recovery usually calls for a six- to eight-week layoff.*

Stress Fracture

A stress fracture must be distinguished from other causes of "shinsplints," as repeated force across the already damaged bone could lead to a complete fracture. Treatment consists of icing in the acute stage, rest, anti-inflammatory medication and cessation of running that causes pain. Placement in a cast is usually not required. (See section on stress fracture in Chapter 5.)

Treatment of "Runner's Knee"

Treatment of "runner's knee" depends, of course, on the diagnosis. The term "runner's knee" is an imprecise, wastebasket term used to describe any pain in the knee that occurs in a runner. It has no medical meaning. Appropriate treatment demands an accurate diagnosis by a knowledgeable physician. Medical science and common sense have much to offer a runner with knee problems. The following are the options open to any individual. These are covered in more detail in specific chapters of this book.

Treatment Options for Knee Pain

1. Rest
2. Decrease mileage
3. Change running shoes
4. Change running surface or terrain
5. Change training program
6. Stretching exercises
7. Knee braces
8. Anti-inflammatory medications
9. Cortisone injections
10. Physical therapy
11. Ice
12. Heat and ultrasound
13. Electrical stimulation
14. Surgery

The best therapy is to prevent a problem before it starts. Training should proceed in an orderly fashion with a gradual increase in distance. An adequate warm-up period is one of the most important and fundamental requirements, particularly for persons with tight hamstrings or problem Achilles tendons. Many runners with inflammation problems find that taking aspirin or other anti-inflammatory medications before and after jogging is quite helpful. Icing the painful area immediately after a long run may also be beneficial. All individuals are not physiologically capable of comparable running accomplishments. Each person must find the appropriate terrain, distance, interval, and training program which serves his needs and does not cause any bodily harm.

This description of runners' injuries has admittedly been brief, and all possibilities have not been covered. If you receive just one message from this chapter, it should be that the knee is a highly complex system with a potential for derangements in many places. Pain that does not go away reasonably quickly should be evaluated by your physician so that worse problems may be prevented. Sometimes, very simple modifications of a running program may produce dramatic results and prevent conditions which would otherwise require extensive and lengthy rehabilitation and treatment.

Children and Running

The growing American concern with fitness is being conveyed to children who are participating in organized sports and running in increasing numbers. More than 20 million children are part of organized athletics of some sort, and millions of others run or jog regularly.

Children derive enormous benefit from athletics and running, not only in physical development, but also in a sense of accomplishment, teamwork and friendship. This early training should lead to a life of healthful exercise habits. Whether this early exercising will ultimately lead to increased longevity and better health is a question only long-term studies will be able to answer, even though such a conclusion seems logical.

There are, however, drawbacks to strenuous athletic performance. Children are often pushed beyond their capabilities by parents who see in their children an opportunity for achievement and notoriety they were never able to accomplish. Likewise, coaches, in their pursuit of victory, place monumental pressures on young children, often in the guise of team spirit and discipline. What should be fun and enjoyable is not.

Young bodies, both physically and psychologically, are often not capable of withstanding the stresses of competitive sports without problems. Children are currently developing overuse syndrome and stress fractures in unprecedented and alarming numbers.

In regards to running, the American Academy of Pediatrics has issued the following statement: ". . . there exist reports on a limited number of patients that have suggested that children may acquire heel cord injuries, epiphyseal growth plate injuries, and other chronic joint trauma from long-distance running. Children have been shown to tolerate hypothermia or hyperthermic environmental extremes poorly during training or long-distance running. Psychological problems can result from unrealistic goals for distance running by children. Long distance competitive running events, primarily designed for adults, are not recommended for children prior to physical maturation. Under no circumstances should a full marathon (26.2 miles) be attempted by immature youths. After pubertal development is complete, guidelines for adult distance running are appropriate."

When it comes to running, children are not little adults. Let them be children.

10

ARTHRITIS OF THE KNEE

The term **arthritis** literally means "inflammation of a joint." There are more than 100 different kinds of arthritis, but all may cause joint deformity and stiffness through deterioration of cartilage. The arthritis may affect only one or many joints and may involve other connecting tissues and organs in the body. In Great Britain the term "rheumatism" has been used to describe many aches and pains in the body, including those in the joints. However, in the United States the term "arthritis" is more common. Approximately one of every seven individuals in the United States is affected by arthritis, many of these cases involving the knee. Diseases such as rheumatoid arthritis, gout and infectious arthritis are quite common. The most common, however, is degenerative or osteoarthritis in which the joint is literally worn away.

Because there are so many different kinds of arthritis, physicians tend to group them according to their basic mechanism of action:

1. Inflammatory arthritis. In this type, the destruction of the joint is caused by inflammation producing chemicals which erode the joint surface. Rheumatoid arthritis is a classic example.

2. Degenerative arthritis. This form occurs as the result of a joint wearing out.

3. Crystal arthritis. Some diseases result in the formation of crystals in the joint which cause swelling, pain and, eventually, destruction. Gout is an example of this form of arthritis.

4. Infectious arthritis. An infection can seriously affect a joint, resulting in severe destruction if not treated promptly.

5. Arthritis syndromes. Many diseases affecting the whole body combine with arthritis. In some cases, this involves a cell which becomes deranged and starts attacking the body's own cells, including the cartilage of the joint. Systematic erythematosus is one such disease.

Diagnosis of Arthritis

Diagnosing your particular kind of arthritis is essential if proper treatment is to be applied. This requires a careful evaluation by your physician. An accurate diagnosis is particularly important when the knee is involved, as prompt treatment of many forms of arthritis may prevent progression of the disease and compromise of knee function.

FORMS OF ARTHRITIS

A detailed description of arthritis is beyond the scope of this book. The following are brief descriptions of the major forms of arthritis.

Osteoarthritis

The most common form of arthritis is osteoarthritis, also known as degenerative arthritis. This form of arthritis results from wear and tear and is found with increasing frequency as individuals age. The joints on which people walk, the so-called weight-bearing joints, are generally the most severely affected. Heredity is one factor in the development of arthritis. Individuals with previous fractures, those who are overweight, those who have had previous ligament injuries, and those who place unusual stress across the knee in their occupations or hobbies are more prone to developing knee arthritis.

Treatment of arthritis depends on its severity. Arthritis medications may prove quite helpful for relief of pain. In addition, steps must be taken to relieve stress on the joint. Exercises are prescribed to balance the forces across the joint and often prove surprisingly helpful when the knee is involved. A cane may provide significant relief for some individuals. In advanced cases, surgery may be required. Removal of loose fragments of cartilage and bone, which have been worn away as the result of the arthritis, may prove particularly helpful. The joint may need to be realigned to place more force on that part of the knee still relatively normal. In the most severe cases, replacement of the entire knee may be necessary. With the advent of more advanced surgical techniques, physicians are seeking to determine whether certain procedures should be performed with the hope of preventing further deterioration of the joint. There are many research studies currently being conducted on the precise procedures and the consequences of each. At a more basic level, many scientists are pursuing very sophisticated research on cartilage and bone and why they tend to deteriorate with age in so many people.

For many years, removal of the entire meniscus for a tear was recommended. However, studies began to show that individuals who had a complete meniscectomy were more prone to develop arthritis earlier in their lives on the side on which the meniscus was removed. Therefore, physicians, in general, are now removing only the damaged portion of the meniscus. Further studies on repairs of the meniscus are still being performed. The goal is prevention of osteoarthritis on the affected side of the knee. Much more time will be required to determine the optimal treatment for these injuries.

Rheumatoid Arthritis

Rheumatoid arthritis affects more than 6 million people in our country. In one of five individuals affected, the disease may disappear spontaneously. In others, it may range from a mild kind of arthritis to one which is severe and crippling. The knee is one of

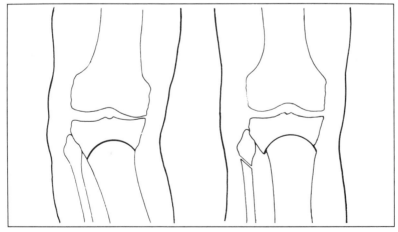

When arthritis has developed on one side of the knee and has left the other side fairly normal, the bone can be cut and the knee realigned to redistribute pressure more evenly.

the most frequently involved joints and, when affected, tends to be particularly painful. Most individuals eventually experience involvement of multiple joints. Other organ systems may also be affected. Initial symptoms may include fever, tiredness, poor appetite, loss of weight and anemia. Involvement of the heart and lungs may cause poor endurance and difficulty breathing. When the skin is affected, an individual may bruise easily and have difficulty with wounds healing. Most commonly, individuals have several attacks of pain and swelling separated by periods of reduced symptoms. In rare cases, there may be a progressive degeneration of joint cartilage.

Treatment consists of control of the inflammation with medication, a specific program of rest and exercise, a carefully designed rehabilitation effort, and, in many cases, splints and assistive devices. Aspirin remains the mainstay of drug therapy, although many new medications have also proven effective. A new class of drugs called nonsteroidal, anti-inflammatory medications are helpful for individuals who are not able to tolerate aspirin. Patients who fail to respond to these basic medications may require treatment with more potent drugs such as penicillamine, gold and even cortisone (steroids). These drugs are only used when absolutely necessary—side effects can be severe. Patients taking these medications must be monitored very closely.

Gout

Gout is a disease caused by an overabundance of uric acid. In the past, individuals have often referred to any sudden arthritis as gout. The word itself is derived from Latin and means "a drop." This term reflects an early belief that the disease was caused by a poison falling drop by drop into the joint. Victims of gout have often been individuals of royalty and renown and may even have included Isaac Newton, Charles Darwin, Martin Luther, George IV of England and Benjamin Franklin. For many years, it was common lore that overindulgence of alcohol could trigger attacks, and now there is confirming scientific evidence. A small amount of uric acid is produced by all persons. Some manufacture an excessive amount, while others are unable to excrete even the normal amounts, causing the uric acid to accumulate in the body. A blood test can be performed to detect an increased level of uric acid. An excess amount may cause crystals to form in joints, leading to attacks of pain and swelling.

In more than half of those who have gout, the initial attack involves the great toe—a condition known as podagra. Virtually any joint may be affected, but the knee is quite commonly involved. To determine whether an individual has gout, uric acid crystals must be seen in the fluid removed from the inflamed joint.

Fortunately, gout is now treatable. The medication allopurinol (Zyloprim) is able to prevent the accumulation of uric acid in the body. In other cases, when crystals form, anti-inflammatory medications, such as colchicine, phenylbutazone (Butazolidin), and indomethacin (Indocin) are quite effective in controlling attacks. The medication probenacid (Benemid) can also be effective in preventing attacks in certain individuals. Because there are multiple causes of gout, it is important to have a thorough medical evaluation to determine the specific abnormality before treatment is begun.

Treatment of Arthritis

The most important part of treatment is early recognition of the problem. Proper treatment of an unstable knee may prevent future problems. For many forms of arthritis, there is no cure, but the disease may often be controlled or slowed. Treatment consists of many facets that may include (1) exercises, (2) medication, (3) skills for protecting a damaged joint, (4) surgery, (5) braces and (6) modification of activities. Beware of those who offer you a guaranteed or instant cure, often without even knowing your kind of arthritis. There are legions of charlatans and swindlers who prey on people in pain. There is a saying in medicine that "The physician who treats himself has a fool for a doctor." This statement may be even more accurate for an arthritis sufferer who attempts to diagnose and treat his own ailment.

FOR MORE INFORMATION

If you have further questions about arthritis, (1) ask your physician; (2) contact the local chapter of the Arthritis Foundation; or (3) write to the national office of the Arthritis Foundation. This organization is a valuable source of information. If you write them, they will take the time to answer your questions. They will also be able to supply you with information on all aspects of arthritis care and treatment

Address: *The Arthritis Foundation*
1314 Spring St. NW
Atlanta, GA 30309

11

MEDICATIONS FOR THE KNEE

Many medications are frequently prescribed by physicians during the course of treatment of knee injuries and arthritis. The purpose of this chapter is to provide a brief understanding of some of these medications so that they can be appropriately used. Only basic medications will be covered, divided into five classes:

1. Aspirin and other salicylates
2. Nonsteroidal, anti-inflammatory drugs (NSAID)
3. Medication for muscle soreness and spasm
4. Pain medications
5. Rubs

ASPIRIN

Aspirin is the most widely used drug in the world. More than 100 million pills are consumed daily. Aspirin has four primary effects:

- relief of pain (analgesic)
- reduction of fever (anti-pyretic)
- prevention of blood clots (anti-phlebitic)
- reduction of inflammation (anti-inflammatory)

Arthritis depends not only on aspirin's analgesic or painkilling effect but, most importantly, on its ability to reduce swelling and inflammation. At the dosage normally taken, aspirin acts only as a painkiller. An individual must take 9 to 20 tablets of five grains each for an anti-inflammatory effect. A standard aspirin tablet contains five grains (325 mg). There appears to be little therapeutic difference between the high-priced, name-brand aspirin and other brands.

The most severe complications from taking aspirin are gastrointestinal. Ulcers have been reported, and patients have also noted nausea, vomiting and ringing in the ears. This latter symptom may indicate that the dosage is too high. Taking the drug with food or antacids may protect the stomach from some of the side effects. For some individuals, coated aspirin has proved quite helpful. In rare cases, a person may develop an allergy to aspirin, indicated by a rash, runny nose, wheezing or shock. If an individual has any new problems after taking aspirin, a physician should be notified.

Aspirin may increase the effect of blood clotting medications, diabetes drugs, insulin, cortisone, anti-seizure medications and sulfa antibiotics. Large doses of vitamin C may cause a toxic level of aspirin to develop.

NONSTEROIDAL ANTI-INFLAMMATORY MEDICATIONS

These medications are a newly developed class of arthritis drugs often capable of controlling the swelling, tenderness and pain of arthritis without the serious side effects of the steroid type of drug. They seem to act by reducing the levels of a substance called prostaglandin. The drugs are used primarily by individuals with rheumatoid arthritis and osteoarthritis, but they may be effective for any condition in which there is inflammation.

The following table lists the nonsteroidal anti-inflammatory medications currently available in this country:

Drug	Chemical Name	Tablet Size	Usual Dosage/Day
Anaprox	Naproxen Sodium	275 mg	4 tablets
Butazolidin	Phenylbutazone	100 mg	4 tablets
Clinoril	Sulindac	150, 200 mg	2 tablets
Indocin	Indomethacin	25, 50 mg	4 tablets
Meclomen	Meclofenamate	50, 100 mg	4 tablets
Motrin	Ibuprofen	400, 600 mg	4 tablets
Nalfon	Fenoprofen	300, 600 mg	4 tablets
Naprosyn	Naproxen	250, 375 mg	2 tablets
Rufen	Ibuprofen	400 mg	4 tablets
Tandearil	Oxyphenbutazone	100 mg	3 tablets
Tolectin	Tolmetin	200, 400 mg	4 tablets

The primary complications of this group of drugs are gastrointestinal. Patients have reported abdominal pain, dyspepsia, nausea, diarrhea, constipation, rashes, dizziness, headaches, and swelling. An individual who has any new problems after taking a medication should notify his physician. Persons taking these medications should also tell their physicians about any other drugs they are concurrently taking.

MEDICATIONS FOR MUSCLE SORENESS AND SPASM

Flexoril (Cyclobenzaprine)

Flexoril is an anti-spasm medication used (along with rest and physical therapy) to relieve muscle spasms caused by acute conditions. It is not effective for treatment of arthritis or inflammations. The use of Flexoril for longer than two or three weeks is not recommended. Flexoril may impair the physical or mental abilities required to perform hazardous tasks such as operating machinery or driving a motor vehicle. A person with urinary retention, glaucoma or heart disease or who is taking drugs for depression must exercise particular caution when taking this medication. You should never drink alcohol when using Flexoril. Forty percent of persons using Flexoril report some nasal dryness. A dry mouth, dizziness, increased heart rate, weakness and fatigue are also commonly reported side effects.

Norgesic (Orphenadrine Citrate)

Norgesic, an analgesic or painkiller used to relieve mild to moderate musculoskeletal pain, is not effective for treatment of arthritis. Patients are warned that Norgesic may impair ability to perform potentially hazardous activities such as operating machinery or motor vehicles. Persons with ulcers, those who have clotting difficulty, or who take aspirin should exercise caution when using Norgesic. Individuals with glaucoma, prostate disease, myasthenia gravis or sensitivity to aspirin or caffeine should not take this drug. Long-term use may cause gastrointestinal disturbances, anemia and kidney damage. Common side effects include a rapid heartbeat, dry mouth, blurred vision, weakness and skin rashes.

Soma (Carisoprodol)

Soma is a muscle relaxant used along with rest, physical therapy and other measures to relieve the discomfort of acute, painful musculoskeletal conditions. It is not useful for treatment of arthritis and inflammatory conditions. Performance of potentially hazardous tasks such as driving a motor vehicle or operating machinery may be impaired by this drug. Persons with acute intermittent porphyria or an allergy to this drug or related compounds such as Meprobamate (Miltown) should not take Soma. Depressants—either drugs or alcohol—should never be taken at the same time. Persons with liver or kidney disease should exercise particular care. Side effects include drowsiness, dizziness, headache, tremor, and skin rash.

Parafon Forte (Chlorzoxazone and Acetaminophen)

Parafon Forte is an analgesic or painkiller used along with rest and physical therapy to relieve the discomfort associated with musculoskeletal conditions. It is not an anti-inflammatory agent and has no effect on arthritis or inflammation. Persons with liver disease should take this medication with caution and should never drink alcohol while taking it. The effect of the drug may be increased if depressants are taken simultaneously. Drowsiness, dizziness, lightheadedness and bleeding under the skin are some side effects.

Quinam (Quinine Sulfate)

Quinam is a muscle relaxant used to treat muscle cramps that occur in the leg at night. Individuals with arthritis, diabetes, varicose veins and vein inflammation seem to be prone to these cramps. Persons with a sensitivity to quinine or those who have a blood defect known as G6PD deficiency should not take Quinam. Individuals taking blood thinners should be particularly careful, as well as those who have ringing in their ears or who have had black water fever. Side effects include ringing in the ears, dizziness, decreased tearing, skin rash, and visual disturbances. Quinam may increase the effects of digitalis medications.

Robaxin (Methocarbamol)

Robaxin is an analgesic or painkiller used along with rest, physical therapy and other measures to relieve the pain and discomfort associated with musculoskeletal conditions. It is not an anti-inflammatory medication and is not effective for the treatment of arthritis. The drug should not be taken by an individual who has had a previous reaction to it. Persons with epilepsy, myasthenia gravis or kidney disease may be sensitive to Robaxin. A combination pill, Robaxisal, contains aspirin, so persons with ulcers or those taking blood thinners should not take this medication. The drug may cause sedation and should not be taken by those participating in hazardous activities such as driving or operating machinery. Alcohol increases the sedative effect. Lightheadedness, lethargy, drowsiness and skin rashes are some of the side effects.

Valium (Diazepam)

Valium is a tranquilizer used to relieve skeletal muscle spasms caused by local injuries. It can also be used to relieve spasticity, anxiety, tension and the symptoms associated with acute alcohol withdrawal and seizures. Valium acts on the central nervous system and serves ultimately as a depressant. It is one of the most misused and overprescribed medications in America. Individuals who are sensitive to Valium or who have glaucoma should not take this medication. When taking Valium, caution should be exercised while operating machinery, driving a motor vehicle or where mental alertness is required. Valium may produce physical or psychological dependence and trigger seizures when it is discontinued. It should be used with caution in combination with other depressants and sedatives, particularly alcohol. Drowsiness, lethargy, skin rash, dizziness, fainting and hallucinations are some of the possible side effects.

PAIN MEDICATIONS

Pain medications should be used judiciously as they tend to mask pain and may lead to overuse of an irritated or inflamed joint. Pain medications, other than anti-inflammatory drugs, do nothing to reduce inflammation. Longterm use of pain medications, particularly narcotics, will cause the body to develop a tolerance and render them less effective. Narcotics are, in addition, potentially addictive.

Dolobid (Diflunisal)

Dolobid is an analgesic painkiller with nonsteroidal, anti-inflammatory properties. It is used to relieve moderate pain of the musculoskeletal system. Dolobid should not be used by persons who have shown previous sensitivity to it or in whom acute asthma attacks, hives, or runny nose have developed following the use of aspirin or other nonsteroidal, anti-inflammatory drugs (NSAIDs). It must be used with caution by persons with ulcers, kidney disease, heart disease, high blood pressure, or a tendency for fluid retention. The side effects of Dolobid are similar to the NSAIDs.

Tylenol, Datril, Phenaphem (Acetaminophen)

Acetaminophen is an analgesic (painkiller) and an anti-pyretic (lowers fever). It is often used in combination with many other medications. Acetaminophen is a relatively safe painkiller but, unlike aspirin, has no anti-inflammatory properties and is not effective for treatment of arthritis and inflammation. It does, however, cause less irritation to the stomach than aspirin when used for treatment of mild pain. Acetaminophen should be taken cautiously by persons with liver or kidney disease. Adverse reactions are infrequent but include drowsiness, skin rash and impaired concentration.

Narcotics

Narcotics are potent pain medications used to relieve severe pain. Narcotics have no anti-inflammatory effect and are not used for treatment of arthritis or inflammation. These medications should not be used before an activity that requires mental alertness, such as driving a car or operating machinery. When combined with alcohol, they may depress the function of the heart and lungs. Narcotics have a high potential for abuse and addiction. They have no place in the treatment of chronic pain or arthritic conditions but are more appropriately used for treating an acute injury. The following medications are some of the commonly used narcotics: Codeine (often combined with Acetaminophen), Dilaudid, Percodan, Talwin, Darvon, Dolene, Darvocet, and Demerol.

Steroids

Corticosteroids or "steroids," as they are commonly called, are a class of chemicals that were rightfully hailed as "miracle drugs" following their discovery in the 1950s. For some diseases, these medications were truly lifesaving; for others, they furnished relief previously only imagined. Initial unbridled enthusiasm was, however, tempered by a sober recognition of the serious side effects of these potent chemicals. The power for dramatic improvement was unfortunately accompanied by a potential for considerable harm.

Corticosteroids are naturally occurring hormones produced by the adrenal gland located over each kidney. This gland secretes corticosteroids in response to the chemical ACTH, which is produced by the master pituitary gland in the brain. The ACTH hormone, which is essential to life, helps maintain metabolic stability and protects the body from stress.

The level of cortisone is delicately controlled in the body, even to the extent that there is a natural daily cycle. One of the causes of jet lag may be a disturbance of this daily fluctuation. An insufficient amount of cortisone leads to Addison's disease. President John F. Kennedy suffered from this condition and required supplemental cortisone to maintain his health.

When given as a drug, cortisone stabilizes the cell membranes and decreases inflammation. Cortisone, or one of the many other synthetic compounds, may be administered by pill, by intramuscular injection, or by injection into an affected bursa, tendon sheath or joint. The following are among the many uses for cortisone:

- adrenal insufficiency (Addison's disease)
- severe asthma unresponsive to less potent medications
- severe rheumatoid arthritis resistant to other drugs
- systemic lupus erythematosus
- severe allergies
- allergic eye and blood vessel diseases
- inflammatory musculoskeletal conditions
- inflammatory bowel disease

When cortisone is taken for a long period of time, the body's ability to produce its own hormone is decreased. If a cortisone patient's system is stressed, such as from an injury or an infection, extra cortisone is absolutely essential. Individuals taking cortisone are advised to wear an identification bracelet in case of a serious accident. Prolonged administration may lead to many serious side effects including cataracts, bruising, loss of calcium from the bones (osteoporosis), weak muscles, susceptibility to infections (including tuberculosis), excessive hair, stretch marks on the abdomen, arthritis of the hips (due to loss of blood supply to the bone) or psychosis. Because of these serious side effects, responsible physicians use cortisone only when absolutely necessary. A number of disreputable arthritis clinics in foreign countries dispense cortisone indiscriminately to unsuspecting victims, who, in some cases, report "miraculous cures." This relief may be achieved not only because of cortisone's powerful anti-inflammatory effect, but also from a state of euphoria created by the medication. The relief is short-lived, however, because long-term cortisone therapy eventually will cause detrimental side effects.

Cortisone Injections

Injections of cortisone into the joints of athletes has been one of the saddest chapters in all of American sports. Cortisone, often in combination with the painkiller Xylocaine, is injected into a joint so an athlete can continue to play on a damaged extremity. Although the athlete experiences immediate pain relief, it is at the expense of possible permanent damage to the joint surface. Many athletes have incurred painful arthritis and their careers have been prematurely ended by this inappropriate use of corticosteroids. Fortunately, many athletes, coaches, and physicians are now more sensitive to the consequences of cortisone injection into a joint or tendon, and much more rational use is made of the drug.

When used appropriately, cortisone injections are a valuable treatment option that delivers a powerful anti-inflammatory effect to an inflamed area while minimizing the side effects in the rest of the body. The drug may be injected into any desired area. The most common sites of use are:

1. joints
2. bursa
3. tendon sheaths
4. trigger points

In severe rheumatoid arthritis, injection of cortisone into an inflamed joint diminishes pain and swelling by decreasing synthesis of the potent chemical prostaglandin and controlling certain white cell functions. Repeated injections are not recommended, but an occasional injection may prove very beneficial. There is little evidence, despite many anecdotal reports, that injection of cortisone is of any benefit in treating osteoarthritis. It may bring temporary relief because of its short-term, anti-inflammatory effect, but there is no evidence that cortisone retards joint destruction. On the contrary, some studies (primarily in animals) suggest that repeated injections may accelerate the arthritic process in a weight-bearing joint such as the knee.

In perhaps 2 percent of people whose joints are injected with cortisone, an acute synovitis occurs. The joint becomes very painful and swollen for 12 to 48 hours. The synovitis is a chemical reaction that will resolve spontaneously, but pain medication and ice may be required for control of discomfort. Although injections are generally safe, certain precautions must be followed, and sterile technique must be used. Infection occurs in about one of every 10,000 injections. The following conditions make a cortisone injection hazardous:

1. an infected joint
2. a severe infection elsewhere in the body
3. an infection near the site of injection
4. ulceration of the skin near the injection site
5. an allergy to the cortisone compound
6. a bleeding disorder
7. use of anti-coagulation medication
8. poorly controlled diabetes

Tendinitis and bursitis may improve dramatically with a cortisone injection. If used judiciously with other modes of treatment, including rest, such injections may allow an athlete to achieve his potential. There are dangers, however, with repeated injections of tendons and tendon sheaths. A tendon may be weakened by a partial tear or from chronic inflammation. In these cases, cortisone injection may retard the healing process and lead to a complete rupture of the tendon. Pain relief may also allow a return to strenuous activity before the tendon has had an opportunity to heal adequately, especially in the patellar (knee) or Achilles (heel) tendon of an athlete such as a high jumper, who exerts explosive force across the involved tendon. These tendons should be injected with cortisone only as a last resort.

RUBS AND CREAMS

A vast array of gels, lotions, liniments and ointments are used by individuals for relief of muscular and arthritic pain. There is no convincing scientific evidence that these products in any way affect the course of injury. In many cases, however, individuals who use them report pain relief. These products may seem to work because they contain counter irritant agents which are applied over the skin where there is pain. These counter irritants produce a mild, local, inflammatory action that create a feeling of warmth and tingling in the skin. Many theories have been proposed as to exactly why the medications seem to work. An individual's attention may be diverted from the underlying pain in the joint, and the stimulation from the skin may change the perception of the brain to other stimuli from the same area of the body. The small blood vessels in the skin are dilated, and the blood flow to the skin is increased as a result of these medications. Burns may result if they are used in combination with a heating pad.

The primary agents in rubs and creams are: methyl salicylate, which occurs naturally as wintergreen or sweet birch oil; camphor, a mild local anesthetic; menthol, which is found naturally as Japanese mint oil; and thymol. These substances can be extremely toxic if ingested, and death may result if as little as one teaspoonful is consumed by a child. They are intended for use on intact skin. If applied to broken skin or an open sore, they may reach toxic levels in the bloodstream.

DMSO

Dimethyl sulfoxide (DMSO) is a simple, naturally occurring organic compound which has generated a storm of controversy and publicity because some claim it qualifies as a wonder drug. There have been reports that this drug has been effective in treating sports injuries, osteoarthritis, rheumatoid arthritis, gout, viruses, burns, parasites and even mental conditions. Its use is advocated by some people for treatment of overuse syndromes caused by running.

DMSO is a byproduct of the paper industry and has been used for many years as an industrial solvent. It has the unusual ability to penetrate the intact skin. In the early 1960s, many experiments were performed using this drug, and perhaps 100,000 patients had received DMSO by 1965. However, studies disclosed damage to the eyes of dogs, rabbits and pigs that were administered DMSO. Although this complication was not observed in humans, distribution of the medication was discontinued by the Food and Drug Administration. The possibility of eye damage in humans still remains a questionable consequence of using DMSO. The drug was discontinued not only because of the side effects, but because there is still no convincing evidence, as a result of controlled scientific testing, to indicate that DMSO is effective for the treatment of musculoskeletal pain.

Many scientific investigations are currently being performed to evaluate DMSO. Presently, the medication is approved only for the treatment of a very rare bladder disorder called interstitial cystitis. Unfortunately, many profiteers are capitalizing on the fanfare surrounding DMSO.

DMSO is generally available in four strengths. The 50 percent strength is used for treating the bladder condition. The 70 percent concentration is the type generally used by physicians for controlled studies. A 90 percent concentration of DMSO is used by veterinarians for treating acute swelling caused by trauma in horses and dogs. A 100 percent solution is available as an industrial solvent and, unfortunately, this product is most frequently used by individuals to treat painful conditions. There is no guarantee of purity with this product, and DMSO may carry impurities into the body not only from itself, but from the skin as well. The reactions to application of DMSO on the skin include redness, itching, a generalized skin rash and a garlic-like taste and odor on the breath occurring a few minutes after administration. A recent study found that tendons were weakened as a result of treatment with DMSO.

In summary, if you choose to use DMSO, you may be exposing yourself to unknown risks from a chemical whose effectiveness is unconfirmed.

OVER-THE-COUNTER PAIN MEDICATIONS

An extraordinary variety of pain medications is available without a prescription. Many of these medicines are advertised frequently in the media and are recommended for virtually all types of human pain. Choosing the least expensive drug appropriate for your problem can be difficult and can actually be a hazard to your health. Many of these medications contain not just one drug but a combination. One of the dangers of multiple medicines in one pill is inadvertent exposure to a drug to which you may be sensitive or allergic. Read the label on the bottle carefully, particularly if there have been any drug reactions or problems which could be made worse with certain drugs (an ulcer, for instance).

Most over-the-counter medications contain a combination of aspirin, caffeine, acetaminophen (Tylenol), and salicylamide. The chemical phenacetin was previously a component of many pills but has been removed from most medications due to potentially serious side effects.

Aspirin, in the doses recommended, is effective for relief of pain and fever. It is not prescribed for relief of inflammation when combined with other drugs. A person taking aspirin or a nonsteroidal, anti-inflammatory drug (NSAID) should avoid any additional medicines which contain aspirin, to avoid producing a toxic dose. (See aspirin section for more detailed information.)

Choline salicylate is a compound related to aspirin and is available in liquid form. Salicylamide is structurally similar to aspirin but is inferior for most uses. The Food and Drug Administration advisory panel on non-prescription drugs says that ". . . it is probably ineffective in the recommended dose...when used as a single analgesic."

Acetaminophen is a relatively safe medication, although an inadvertent overdosage can cause serious, even fatal, liver damage. It is effective for pain and fever, but has no effect on inflammation. A person should not take it in hopes of relieving the pain and swelling of arthritis.

Caffeine is commonly used in combination with aspirin and acetaminophen. Many people are sensitive to caffeine. Too much can cause irregular heartbeats, sleeplessness and nervousness.

Sodium, often in large quantities, is a common component of over-the-counter medications for pain relief. Many people are prone to retain fluid and elevate their blood pressure if they consume too much sodium.

Each of these medications has multiple effects and side effects plus reactions with other drugs. When your physician asks you what medications you are taking, be sure to include any that you buy on your own.

12

EXERCISES FOR THE KNEE

"**O**f all the** methods of alleviating and even curing many infirmities to which the body is subject, there is nothing to equal exercise. Rest has its advantages—it repairs dissipated spirits and refreshes the fatigued body. It helps to cure many diseases; but under this pretext, to refrain from all exercise is a great error...let us remember that the abuse of rest is more dangerous than that of exercise." Nicolas Andry, M.D., French physician, 1723.

Proper functioning of the knee requires adequate and appropriate training of the leg muscles. This training includes not only those muscles which are attached to the knee itself but also those which supply power to the ankle and the hip. The knee is essential for supporting the body, stabilizing the leg, and propelling an individual to achieve motion. All of these functions depend upon a coordinated effort by the muscles of the leg.

Exercises should be specifically tailored to an individual's problems and needs. There are many different types of exercises. Performing the wrong exercises may be inefficient and a waste of time and, in some cases, may even be harmful. For instance, a marathon runner training to increase his endurance or a football player exercising to develop strength, requires vastly different exercise programs from a recreational athlete who has undergone surgery and now needs to rehabilitate his knee. In addition, individuals who have sustained a ligament injury or who have had surgical repair of a ligament require very specific exercise and rehabilitation programs that will not only strengthen their weakened muscles, but to protect the newly repaired ligaments until sufficient strength has been regained.

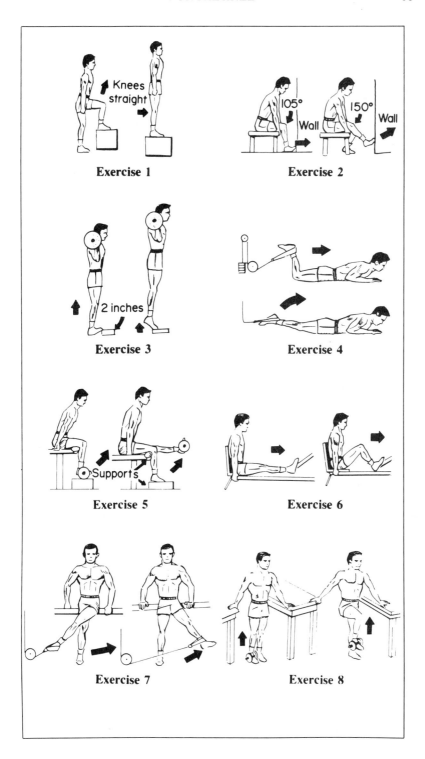

Exercise 1

Exercise 2

Exercise 3

Exercise 4

Exercise 5

Exercise 6

Exercise 7

Exercise 8

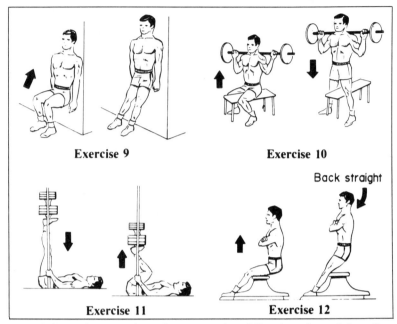

Exercise 9   Exercise 10

Exercise 11   Exercise 12

*West Point cadets are given these exercises following a knee injury. Specific exercises are recommended depending on the injury. (From **Treatment of Injuries to Athletes**, 4th ed. by Don O'Donoghue, W.B. Saunders Co., Philadelphia, 1984, with permission)*

A weakened lower extremity is more susceptible to injury. The conditioning of the muscles should be appropriate to the stress which will be placed on them. The requirements depend not only on the demands of the sport, but also on the condition of the knee. A previously damaged knee may require special conditioning to compensate for that injury. Thus, exercises are performed to: 1) maintain normal muscular strength; 2) rehabilitate the musculature of the leg following an injury; 3) develop muscular capacity specific to a desired sport or activity, and 4) protect the knee from injury.

The Function of Exercise

Exercises serve seven basic functions:

1. Strength
2. Endurance
3. Range of motion or flexibility
4. Cardiovascular improvement
6. Weight maintenance
7. Sense of well-being

Each individual, in pursuing an exercise program, must determine his priorities and goals before selecting the appropriate program. Exercises performed slowly to gain motion or flexibility may provide no help in achieving strength or in developing a specific skill for a sport. Likewise, those performed for endurance may lead to very little increase in strength.

No one exercise will achieve all of an individual's goals. This simple fact is often forgotten when criticizing some regimens that do not meet goals for which they were never intended. To achieve the multiple performance goals, multiple exercises must be practiced.

The Basics

The development of skills for recreation and sport requires much more than just strength building. Muscles are ultimately responsible for moving a joint. However, this motion must be orchestrated by the brain and peripheral nervous system to produce the desired motion. Muscle fibers must be stimulated to contract in a smooth and coordinated pattern if the body is to function properly. Failure to achieve this coordinated motion results in jerky, often uncontrolled, irregular movements which, when severe, are referred to as "spastic." To accomplish a controlled motion, some muscles must be stimulated to pull an extremity in one direction (referred to as the agonist) while muscles which pull the extremity in the opposite direction (antagonist) must be relaxed. This extraordinary coordination, in most cases, occurs automatically without conscious thought. There is an awareness of this complex interaction only when it malfunctions. Some people seem to have a more efficient nervous system than others and are able to activate or recruit more of their muscle fibers.

A determined attitude is also a vital part of muscular performance and is a crucial component in achieving a particular athletic feat. Witness the heroic acts of strength reported by average people when faced with imminent danger. They are stimulating far more of their available fibers and generating more muscular power than is normally available. In addition, exercising only one leg often results in improved strength in the other, a consequence of learning (and neurological efficiency), not muscle conditioning.

Muscle

Muscle is the tissue in the body responsible for motion. Individual muscles are composed of fibers called myofibrils. In turn, each of these myofibrils contains contractile proteins called actin and myosin. Electrical signals from the nervous system cause groups of myofibrils to contract. Each of these groups is referred to as a motor unit. In any one muscle, only select groups of myofibrils are stimulated at any one time. This capability gives human muscle the capacity to contract slowly, in a controlled manner, or explosively, in a very powerful manner.

There are basically two different kinds of muscle fibers: type 1 and type 2. Studies have found a correlation between the predominant fiber type and some types of athletic performance. The type 1 red muscle fibers, also called slow-twitch fibers, are used primarily for activities that demand a continuous supply of oxygen (aerobic). These fibers do not fatigue easily and are the ones most responsible for endurance activities. A marathon runner tends to have a high percentage of type 1 fibers for endurance. The type 2 muscle fiber, or white muscle, is also called a fast-twitch fiber. These muscles are used for very rapid motion, but they fatigue easily and function anaerobically (without oxygen). A sprinter tends to have a predominance of type 2 muscle fibers in those muscles used in running.

Each of us is born with a genetic makeup of muscle fiber type which gives certain innate potential. Although muscle fibers may hypertrophy or grow, there is no scientific evidence that humans can change muscle type, which lends scientific credence to the observation that an individual is born to perform a certain type of athletic activity if he develops his potential. For example, some individuals, no matter how much they exercise, will never develop bulging muscles.

Whenever an extremity is immobilized, such as in a cast, or on crutches, muscles tend to atrophy (or waste away). Type 1 fibers seem to atrophy the quickest, but with prolonged rest, both types of fibers show considerable atrophy. Individuals who are taking corticosteroids (steroids) seem to have a particular tendency for atrophy of type 2 fibers.

Ironically, one of the dangers of prolonged space flight is weightlessness, which removes all stress from bones and muscles. Bones and muscles require continued stress to maintain their normal structure and function. Early astronauts developed severe muscle weakness when an adequate exercise program was not performed in space. Now, spacecraft used for prolonged flights are equipped with exercise devices so astronauts can maintain their muscular strength, coordination and endurance as much as possible in weightlessness.

As training has become more scientific, athletic trainers, physical therapists and physicians have recommended exercises to improve performance in a particular type of event and to improve hypertrophy (growth) of one fiber type. Marathon runners train using exercises that have been shown to develop type 1 fibers, while high jumpers do exercises demonstrated to result in growth of type 2 fibers. Routine muscle biopsies of athletes in this country have not been established. In some countries, however, individuals are tested at a young age, and based on the results of muscle biopsies and other tests, such as pulmonary function and cardiovascular endurance, they are groomed and trained for specific sports.

JUDGING MUSCLES

The ultimate test of a muscle's function is its ability to protect a joint and to allow participation at a desired level in a particular activity. Great demands are made upon individual muscles, and scientists have found assessment of muscle function, as it relates to performance, to be somewhat difficult because of the multiple capacities of the neuromuscular system.

Strength

Strength is an objective performance measure, although it is defined in various ways and measured by many different techniques. Strength could be defined as the ability to develop a force against unyielding resistance. In this way, strength can be assessed as the ability to lift a certain weight or the ability to apply a certain force to an object. When this force is applied as an object rotates around an axis, which is really the situation when the leg rotates around the knee, the term "torque" is used. Torque represents the force applied times the distance from the axis.

Power

The ability to develop power is one of the most important capacities of muscle. Power is a term derived from physics and represents the ability to do work at a certain rate. It is a measure not only of strength or the ability to develop a force, but also the ability to sustain that force while the muscle shortens or lengthens. In strict terms, power is defined as the force a muscle develops times its velocity or how quickly it moves (shortens or lengthens). There is considerable variation in power from individual to individual. A person who is able to generate a significant force may not be able to maintain that force in a rapid powerful fashion useful for a particular event. Of course, that explains some of the great differences in individual abilities in various sporting events

Flexibility

Flexibility is an important factor in assessing joint function. The range of motion of a joint determines its flexibility. The ability to extend the knee is vitally important for efficient functioning of the leg. An individual should be able to flex or bend the knee to about 80 degrees for normal walking, and an additional 10 to 20 degrees to climb stairs normally.

Physicians treating a knee injury frequently begin with what are called "range of motion" exercises—specific exercises whose goal is to increase the ability of the joint to move. For the knee, this method is particularly important to regain normal function.

There are two types of range of motion exercises: 1) active and 2) passive. In an active exercise, the individual provides the muscle power for movement of the joint through its range. When a therapist or trainer assists with this motion, the exercise is referred to as an "active-assisted" exercise. In the passive type of exercise, a therapist or trainer moves the joint through its range. If there is severe weakness or if there is pain with contraction of a muscle, the joint can be kept mobile and a contracture prevented. When there has been a ligament repair, passive range of motion is often employed so the joint remains mobile but excessive stress is not placed across a healing ligament. Maintaining motion in a joint is important to preserve healthy cartilage. Unfortunately, no muscular strength is gained with the passive range of motion.

There is a natural tendency for a person whose knee is painful and swollen to keep the joint in a flexed position, and there are often muscle spasms following an injury. Such flexion for short periods of time will generally not cause any problems; however, if the flexion is maintained, a permanent contracture may develop and prevent the individual from straightening his knee. Particularly when arthritis is involved, an individual who develops a contracture in his knee may be creating an irreversible condition which will lead to compromise of his ability to walk normally and participate in many activities.

Endurance

Endurance, the ability to sustain muscular force, is likewise a vitally important aspect of muscular function. In general, endurance depends not only on the ability of the muscle, but also on the cardiovascular and nutritional system to continue to supply the muscle with the necessary oxygen and nutrients. Training for endurance generally requires multiple repetitions with low resistance to achieve improvement.

Warm-up Exercises

Before beginning any strenuous activity or demanding exercise, you should warm up to gradually stretch the involved muscles, tendons, ligaments and capsule to prevent injury. Athletes have learned that stretching is essential to avoid injury. Pulled

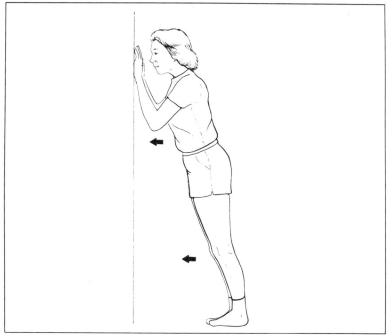

Here's a stretch for the Achilles tendon. Place your feet together about two feet from a wall. Lean forward and brace yourself against the wall. Don't stretch so much as to cause pain.

hamstring muscles and cramps in the calf are often the result of an inadequate warmup. Heat may also prove valuable: preparing muscles for vigorous activity. Individuals who are not naturally

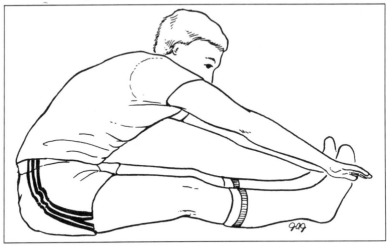

This is a stretch for the hamstrings and lower back. Lean forward with your arms outstretched and try to touch your toes.

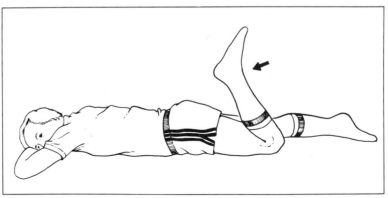

To stretch the quadriceps muscles, lie face down and bend a leg at the knee. Try to touch your heel to your buttocks.

loose or who are injured should be particularly encouraged to pursue a rigorous warmup. When the Achilles tendon is tight, do deep-knee bends and lean against a wall (feet flat and two feet away) to help loosen the back of the calf. Bending the knee and grabbing the toes near the back of the thigh with a gradual pull encourages motion, not only in the knee, but also in the hip. Lying on the back and grasping the hands around a flexed knee is an excellent exercise for flexing both the hip and the knee. Standing on the toes not only encourages motion of the ankle but also provides stimulation to the posterior calf muscles and stretches the muscles on the front of the leg.

Fine Tuning Performance

Highly sophisticated techniques are now being applied to athletic performance to analyze the components of motion. These procedures enable physicians to identify problem areas and prescribe training and rehabilitative techniques to improve performance. These techniques are applied not only to athletes, but also to people with arthritis and various complex medical conditions with muscular and neurologic abnormalities. Transducers enable scientists to assess the forces applied by an extremity while computers and high-speed photography and video recorders enable scientists to assess speed, acceleration, and patterns of motion. Gait laboratories, as well as laboratories directed at athletic performance, are furnishing a new level of sophistication which enables physicians and trainers to direct their efforts at very specific aspects of human performance.

TYPES OF EXERCISE

There are three basic classes of strengthening exercise:
1. Isometric
2. Isotonic
3. Isokinetic

Isometric Exercises

An isometric exercise is one in which a muscle is contracted without moving the extremity, thus maintaining the joint in a fixed position. Placing the leg against the floor and contracting the quadriceps muscle to its maximum is an example of an isometric exercise of the quadriceps muscle with the joint in full extension. Sitting on the edge of a chair with a belt tied around the ankle and the chair leg and attempting to straighten the leg would similarly be an isometric contraction with the joint held at 90 degrees of flexion. Isometric training has been around for a long time but first became popular in the 1950s. This popularity was based on research which made the rather dramatic claim that a maximum strengthening effect could be achieved by merely contracting a muscle for six seconds at two-thirds of its maximum power. Adherents to this philosophy claimed that the rigorous, repetitive and taxing effort required by traditional weightlifting was needless. Years of subsequent scientific research have not supported this very optimistic claim for strengthening. However, research has established some appropriate areas for isometric strengthening exercises.

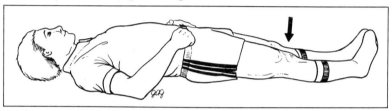

An isometric exercise for the quadriceps calls for lying on your back and pushing your knees toward the floor. Hold for five seconds and then relax your leg muscles.

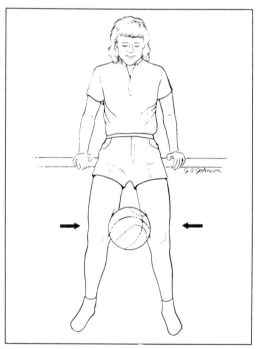

To work the adductor muscles of the leg, try this unique exercise. Place a basketball, soccer ball or similarly sized ball, between your legs and squeeze for five seconds.

One particular benefit of isometric exercises, particularly for arthritis patients, is that the muscles may be stressed without the necessity of moving a painful or inflamed joint. In addition, individuals whose limbs must be immobilized in a cast may find these exercises particularly useful.

The benefits of isometric exercises are the greatest in individuals who have significant weakness. The greatest gains are made during the first month. After that, some studies have found that the strengthening effect is virtually negligible. It would appear from many studies that exercises should be performed daily and should be maximal exercises repeated on many occasions. In addition, if possible, they should be performed with the limb held at varying degrees of flexion, as the maximum strengthening effect appears to be rather specific for the position in which the limb is held.

Isotonic Exercises

The second type of exercise is isotonic (or dynamic). In strict terms, the tension applied to the extremity is constant with this type of exercise. In dynamic exercise, the joint moves through a range of motion against a "constant " resistance. This resistance may take the form of ankle weights or barbells attached to a foot plate or, in other cases, exercise machines may furnish the resistance. In modern times, one of the most influential researchers was Dr. Thomas DeLorme, who, in the 1940s, developed a method known as progressive resistive exercises (PRE). Dr. De-Lorme was an amateur weightlifter who noticed, while he was in the military, that individuals undergoing knee surgery could be restored to strength faster by increasing the resistance of their exercises. At the time, individuals were instructed to do many repetitions using very light weights. He recommended exercising to the point of fatigue until a particular weight was mastered and then increasing the weight to increase the demands. This method produced a progressive increase in strength.

An important concept in isotonic exercise is the repetition maximum, abbreviated RM. A repetition maximum is the ability to lift a certain weight a specific number of times. For instance, a 1 RM weight means an individual can lift that amount of weight only once before he becomes exhausted. A 10 RM weight means an individual can lift that amount of weight 10 times before he reaches exhaustion. Dr. DeLorme initially recommended a rather lengthy routine in which an individual performed 10 sets of exercises starting at a load of one-half of the 10 RM and progressing to the full 10 repetition maximum (10 RM). He subsequently revised this plan so that instead of doing 10 sets of exercise, a person only did three sets. Since his initial pioneering efforts, researchers have tried various permutations and combinations of weights, frequency, number of sets, and duration to achieve the greatest gains in strength. There is a general consensus that the amount of weight necessary to achieve fatigue in five to 10 repetitions may be optimal. The other variations regarding the exercise regimens are not as clear, although scientists are generally in agreement on the basic principle that sufficient tension must be generated by the muscle to overload it.

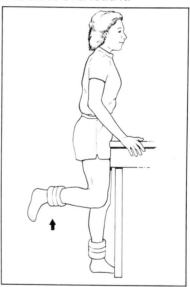

Ankle weights may be used in an isotonic hamstring exercise.

Strength Is Not the Same Everywhere

Due to the mechanics of the knee, individual differences in the attachments of muscles, the different lengths of muscles and the contractile properties of muscle, the knee is not equally strong in all positions. Most individuals can generate the maximum force in extending the knee at approximately 60 degrees. When the knee is bent at a right angle, and when it is nearly straight, the knee is quite weak. When an individual refers to the strength of the knee, the position of the knee must be known to assess just what this means. In addition, because some muscles responsible for straightening or extending the knee are attached to the pelvis, bending the hip up (flexing) will also make a difference: it shortens one of the muscles and actually decreases its ability to straighten the knee. These individual physical differences may lead to significant differences in performance.

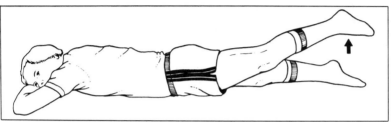

Hamstrings and lower-back strengthening is accomplished by doing this exercise. Lift a leg one foot off the floor and hold it there for about five seconds, lowering slowly. Weights may be added to make the exercise more difficult.

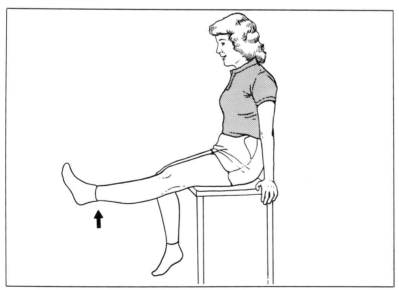

This exercise strengthens the knee and helps improve knee flexibility. While seated, hold a leg straight in front of you for five seconds, then lower slowly.

Concentric vs Eccentric Exercise

If resistance is applied to a muscle as it contracts and shortens, the exercise is referred to as a concentric contraction or positive resistance. If, on the other hand, the resistance is applied and the muscle lengthens, the exercise is considered an eccentric or negative contraction. Both types of exercise are important for increasing the strength capability of a muscle. In the knee, a concentric contraction of the quadriceps muscle occurs when the leg is straightened or extended. An eccentric or negative contraction occurs as the leg is slowly lowered or flexed from a sitting position. Eccentric contractions tend to produce more muscle soreness, particularly if performed precipitously by an untrained individual. Recently, kinesiologists have recognized that running stresses the quadriceps muscle in an eccentric fashion after initial weight bearing; the muscle is lengthening and exerting its high power. The muscle actually absorbs energy from the body to keep the knee from collapsing backwards. Thus, training in which a weight is lifted by the leg but not lowered may not be the optimal method for strengthening this muscle if the goal is improved running performance.

All Weights Are Not the Same

For years, the standard of a knee's strength was the ability to lift a barbell attached to a boot at the foot or a weight attached to a lever of an exercise machine. The barbell is lifted from its resting position (with the leg vertical) as the individual straightens the knee until the leg is parallel with the floor.

Analysis of this system reveals some interesting features of this exercise. A weight hanging on the end of the leg initially causes little resistance to motion, as most of the force from the weight is directed downward and does not resist the motion of the leg. (The force passes through the center of rotation of the knee joint.) This component of resistance gradually increases to a maximum by the time the leg reaches the horizontal position where all of the force of the weight (plus the leg) is perpendicular to the axis of the leg.

The important point of going through this analysis is that even though the weight which hangs on the foot is a constant, the actual resistance to motion is quite different, depending upon the position of the leg. Many different exercise machines are available that generate resistance to motion by a stack of weights. Superficially, they may appear very similar, but the pulley arrangement and the mechanics of a specific exercise machine may result in dramatically different forces being applied to the leg as the joint changes its angle during exercise.

Variable Resistance Exercises

One consequence of the difference in force generated by the knee at different positions is that the limiting factor for determining the greatest weight that can be lifted will be the weakest point of the arc. The muscle will really not be overloaded or stressed at other points, particularly where it is the strongest. In terms of strength development, the muscle will not truly be overloaded throughout its range of motion. The point beyond which a weight cannot be lifted is referred to as the "sticking point." The sticking point is well recognized by weightlifters who perform curls utilizing the biceps muscle.

They often change the angle of the arm, leaning forward or backward, to overcome the sticking point. Another technique used is to rapidly accelerate a weight early in the exercise so that the momentum of the traveling weight will decrease the necessary force required to continue moving the weight upward at other points in the arc.

This shortcoming of barbells, sometimes called fixed weights by some, led to the development of devices called variable resistance exercise machines. The goal of these devices is to apply a resistance or force to the muscle throughout its range of motion which is proportional to the strength of the muscle at that point in the arc. The goal is to promote uniform strengthening of the muscle. Arthur Jones of Nautilus Sports/Medical Industries, Inc. developed a cam-operated exercise machine, now marketed as Nautilus, to apply this adjusted force to the muscle. The applied force to the extremity is based upon an average, determined from deconditioned individuals, which tends to promote a more uniform strengthening of the muscles. According to Nautilus literature, research on this concept and exercise machine began in 1948, although a Nautilus machine was not actually marketed until 1970. The first machine was a pullover torso machine. Nautilus has subsequently marketed an entire line of machines, some for specific muscles of the lower extremity. One particularly valuable feature of the Nautilus exercise machines is the isolation of individual muscles or muscle groups. Traditional exercises with barbells generally require a combination of muscles be brought into play to achieve the desired motion. If one is training for strength, fatigue will occur at the sticking point in the weakest link of the system. The Nautilus equipment, on the other hand, is designed to apply a graded resistance to only one muscular group.

Nautilus equipment is now used in many exercise centers throughout the country and has been an enormous commercial success. The principles of Jones are a definite contribution to exercise physiology and kinesiology. However, a shortcoming of the Nautilus type of equipment is that the torque curves generated are not specific for each individual user but are an approximation of the population. To accommodate the different leg lengths, muscle attachments and muscle strength curves of each individual, a machine specific to each would ideally be required. The theoretical basis of the variable resistance device is compelling, although at present there is limited data available to confirm the effectiveness of the devices and the techniques for achieving improvements in human strength and performance. More time is needed to generate sufficient data to scientifically substantiate this approach as a superior training method.

ISOKINETIC EXERCISES

Isokinetic exercises are performed at a constant speed. "Iso" means "same" and "kinetic" means "motion." These exercises are performed on special equipment on which the speed of movement is a constant, though it can be varied. In fact, the terminology is somewhat confusing in that constant speed refers to angular rotation of the extremity rather than to the linear speed of the muscle. Isokinetic exercises are performed on machines which control the speed of the exercise, keeping it fixed throughout the range of motion as force is applied. The force applied to maintain the range of motion may vary, and therefore the term "accommodating resistance exercise" is used to describe these exercises.

The Cybex and Orthotron, manufactured by Lumex Corp., are examples of isokinetic devices. The first device in modern times was constructed by Perrine in 1965 and has achieved remarkable popularity. In fact, a similar device was constructed 50 years previously for analyzing muscles in a laboratory. An isokinetic device allows an individual to develop muscles at both low and high velocities. Advocates of this method believe that the ability to train at both slow and fast velocities is a desirable feature and enables an individual to strengthen muscles capable of exhibiting both slow and rapid force. Proponents believe this type of exercise is particularly valuable in building power in muscles, enabling them to exert strength at high speeds.

Following its introduction, there was a wave of enthusiasm in which this exercise was labeled "...the most revolutionary form of exercise since Milo." There is some evidence that fast speed isokinetic training may be beneficial for athletes training for sports that require explosive speeds. However, even using high speed training, such machines are inadequate for strengthening ankle plantarflexors (pushing downward) because of the very high velocities and torques required for normal walking, running and jumping. The evidence also seems to indicate that slow-speed isokinetic training is more effective than fast-speed for development of strength. Less muscle soreness seems to be produced using isokinetic training than isotonic exercises. In performing exercises on an isokinetic device, an individual contracts the muscles with a sudden acceleration until contact is achieved with the machine. There is a sudden deceleration during which time the leg slows to match the speed of the bar. Individuals who have recently undergone ligament repair or a total knee joint replacement may sustain injury by this sudden acceleration and deceleration.

Isokinetic devices do result in increases in muscular strength. One disadvantage, particularly for runners who wish to train the quadriceps musculature, is that isokinetic exercise machines furnish only positive exercise training. There is no negative or eccentric training possible on an isokinetic device. Currently, devices manufactured by Lumex Corp. can measure some of the variables of human performance on the Cybex machines. This feature has been particularly helpful in athletics by furnishing an objective measurement of some parameters of performance. There is not universal agreement, however, on the precise meaning of the results of these measurements. The early machines did not correct for the weight of the leg itself, and the results of many studies were inaccurate.

Preventing Injuries While Exercising

One of the primary goals of an exercise program is to furnish the muscle strength and endurance necessary to protect the joint. However, improper performance of an exercise program may actually predispose one to severe injury. To avoid injury, follow these suggestions:

1. *Always warm up* before exerting muscles or performing any physical activity.

2. *Avoid fast, jerky movements* when using weights or exercise machines; the sudden acceleration and deceleration may exceed the capacity of the body's tissues.

3. *Develop muscles in a balanced fashion.* Strengthening one muscle group may expose the knee to injury if the antagonist group of muscles is not similarly developed.

4. *Proceed slowly.* You should proceed in a slow and orderly fashion with any exercise program. Weekend athletes are prone to injury due to excessive stresses placed on an unprepared body.

5. *Stretch before exercising.* Stretching muscles which are going to be used during an exercise will make them less likely to be injured. This practice is particularly important for an individual who naturally has tight muscles such as the hamstrings or the heel cord.

Selecting Your Exercise Program

You must first decide on your goals and recognize your present capabilities before selecting an exercise program. One particular type of exercise will not be adequate for the multi-faceted goals of each individual. For instance, exercise directed at the optimal development of strength may lead to little improvement in cardiovascular function. Performance of a desired activity depends upon many factors. Some are genetic and cannot be altered, while others may respond to an exercise program. Strength and even muscular power are distinct qualities separate from skill. Training may lead to dramatic increases in strength, but improved skill can only result from practice of the specific activity. In a sense, strength may provide potential to achieve a desired activity. Performance depends upon:

1. Strength and power
2. Skill
3. Flexibility
4. Cardiovascular capacity
5. Neurological coordination and efficiency
6. Body mechanics
7. Psychological desire

Exercises may enable a person to attain his maximum capability, but they cannot alter a person's basic body mechanics, innate athletic coordination, muscle fiber type or neurological efficiency. Exercise can, however, increase a muscle's mass or bulk, change the springiness of the muscle and even the percentage area of fast-twitch and slow-twitch fibers by selectively increasing the size of the individual fibers.

Principle of Specificity. Athletes and coaches have found that skills and muscular power developed for one sport may not transfer to another. Patterns of movement, balance, and specific muscular strengths may be quite unique to one particular activity. A javelin thrower may excel at that sport, but may perform very poorly at the shot put, despite the fact that the events are superficially very similar. Likewise, on most professional football teams, the punter is generally different from the placekicker's. Because of these very specific patterns of performance, many believe all training should simulate the movement pattern of the athletic event. The important point to recognize is that skill, agility, and timing result from practice of a particular movement pattern, and that strength is produced by appropriately stressing a muscle. Repetitive performance of an activity (including running) will not lead to significant muscular growth unless the appropriate muscles are overloaded. The two activities are different, and you should try an exercise program which includes both, rather than attempting to find one magic regimen, which may in fact reduce your level of skill.

Stationary Bicycles

Stationary bicycles come in many models, constructed with various degrees of sophistication. The exercise bicycle can be an important part of a knee rehabilitation program. Cycling provides a controlled environment for restoration of muscular strength, endurance and flexibility. The bicycle is particularly valuable for rehabilitation programs following surgery where avoidance of side-to-side stress on the knee is necessary. Successful cycling requires approximately 100 degrees of motion, although raising the seat may allow one to cycle when full motion is not available. When cycling with regular pedals and no toe clips or toe straps, strengthening is restricted primarily to the quadriceps muscles and hip extensor muscles. By using toe clips and straps on the pedals, the hamstrings are strengthened as well. Therefore, for serious rehabilitation, toe clips and straps are essential if one is to sustain a balanced rehabilitative effort. In practice, cycling is probably used more for its beneficial effect on the cardiovascular system than for muscle or joint rehabilitation.

Electrical Stimulation for Muscle Strengthening

In some cases, a muscle is unable to voluntarily contract because of injury to the nerve or, in some cases, because of immobilization in a cast. Electrical stimulation of the muscle has been shown in some studies to aid in strengthening and in preventing atrophy (wasting away) due to inactivity. The use of such devices should always be selective and under the direction of a physician; they should not be used as an easy way of rehabilitating a muscle. These devices are by no means as effective as voluntary and intense contraction of the muscle by an individual.

Specific Exercise Programs

Exercises for patellar problems. Most individuals with patellar problems will respond to a vigorous exercise program, and surgery will not be required. The exercises may be combined with anti-inflammatory medication, protection of the joint from excessive forces, and, occasionally, bracing. The initial goal is to decrease the pain and irritability of the joint with rest and avoidance of activities that place undue force across the joint between the patella and the femur.

Stooping and deep-knee bends are two activities particularly harmful to an individual with patellar problems. In some cases, when the pain is severe, immobilization in a splint may be required. Muscle strengthening exercises are then performed with the knee nearly or fully extended. Initially, a person performs quadriceps setting or isometric exercises. Straight-leg raising exercises are then added.

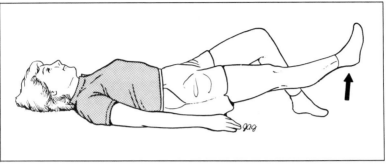

For strengthening muscles in the leg, lie on your back and lift a leg one foot off the floor (measured from the heel). Hold for five seconds and then lower slowly. People with lower-back problems should not do this exercise.

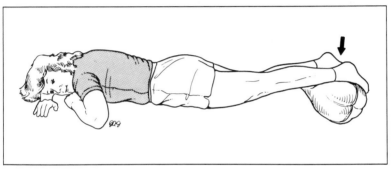

For the quadriceps, lie on your stomach with your ankles supported on a small pillow. Contract the quadriceps muscles, hold for five seconds, relax, then contract again.

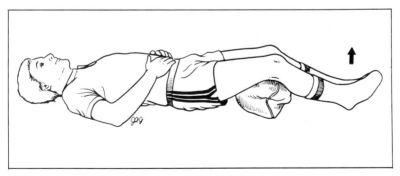

A person with patellar pain and a weak quadriceps is usually started on a short-arc quadriceps exercise to avoid excessive pressure against the undersurface of the kneecap. Straighten the leg and hold for five seconds, then lower slowly.

Following these initial exercises, short arc quadriceps exercises are initiated. These exercises have the distinct advantage that little force is applied between the kneecap and the front of the femur. As strength is gained and pain subsides, weights may be added to accelerate the rehabilitative process. Individuals with patellar problems may actually worsen their condition by doing exercises, particularly with weights in which the knee is flexed more than 30 to 45 degrees. This precaution makes many of the exercises in a standard rehabilitation program inadvisable. It also makes many of the exercise machines potentially harmful if they are not used judiciously. One goal of this exercise program is to selectively strengthen part of the quadriceps muscle called the vastus medialus obliquus, located on the medial or inside of the quadriceps muscle. This muscle is responsible for pulling the kneecap to the midline, stabilizing its travel in the groove on the front of the femur.

Exercises for running. Running is a complex activity which places great demands on the muscular system. In turn, it also produces significant benefits to the body as a whole and to the muscular system in particular. Nevertheless, running is far from a complete and optimal exercise in terms of development of muscular strength, flexibility and endurance.

Research on jogging has revealed some rather fascinating facts: There is now compelling evidence that the calf muscles, responsible for plantarflexing (pushing the ankle down), are the primary source of power in running and are responsible for about 80 percent of the power generated. While not nearly as significant, the muscles of the hip are also responsible for generating power. A most interesting finding has been that the quadriceps muscles contract eccentrically in jogging and, in essence, provide a negative power, as the muscle is contracting maximally during jogging while the knee is bending. The muscles thus serve primarily to prevent the knee from collapsing or bending excessively rather than providing a strong burst of power to straighten the knee, as one would find in a concentric contraction. In terms of rehabilitation and exercise, this finding would seem to indicate that to develop the quadriceps muscles for running, exercises which have both an eccentric (negative) phase and a concentric (positive) phase are likely to be most beneficial. The lowering rather than

lifting of the weight may be the most beneficial. There has probably been an over-reliance in much of the rehabilitation literature
on concentric development of the quadriceps muscle. Clearly,
with the calf muscles providing the primary source of power, the
quadriceps muscles, along with the hamstring muscles and the
muscles of the hip, must be developed to improve performance
in jogging.

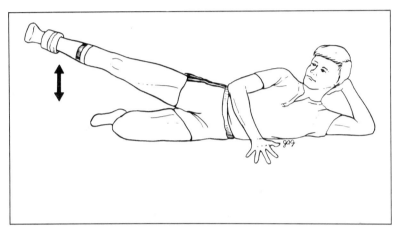

*To work the gluteus medius muscle, lie on your side and lift the upper
leg, keeping it straight. Hold for five seconds, lowering slowly. The hip
abductors are responsible for pulling the hip to the outside or away from
the body.*

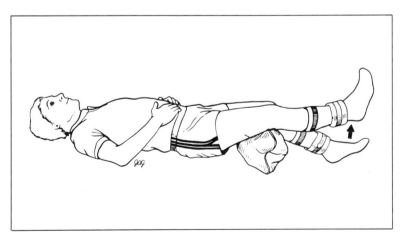

*You may use weights attached to the ankle for the short-arc quadriceps
exercise to increase resistance.*

Organizing an exercise program. The flexibility, strength, endurance and skill for a desired performance are independent to a large extent and demand specific training methods and techniques for improvement. Therefore, while there is certainly crossover from one exercise program to another in terms of benefits, a comprehensive exercise program must involve multiple techniques to achieve a performance goal. Certain exercises must be performed to strengthen desired muscles, while other exercises will create flexibility in certain joints. Skill, including the ability to initiate rapid directional changes (commonly thought of as agility), is attained through training and instruction and is not necessarily related to muscular strength.

It should be obvious that skill in one particular activity is not necessarily transferable to another. Ultimately, performance depends on many factors, some inherited, some created through rigorous training, and some requiring careful instruction and practice. Parts of an exercise program must be specific to the desired performance, but the entire program does not necessarily follow this course.

Movie star exercise programs. We are increasingly besieged by a growing number of exercise programs touted by celebrities. Claims are made for fitness, weight loss and improved well-being. A review of some of these programs reveals that they are helpful because many people who would not typically participate in an exercise program find they enjoy this form of socialized exercising. However, these programs generally have considerable limitations for serious athletes as most of these exercise routines concentrate their musculoskeletal emphasis on flexibility and have very little significant effect on strength development. The rapid, jerky motions recommended by some programs may lead to muscle and ligament tears in the ill-prepared individual due to excessive and sudden overload of the system. Individuals with injured extremities may make their conditions worse by following the typical exercise session. If you do have problems, check with your physician before beginning any exercise program.

PHYSICAL MODALITIES

In addition to exercise, people who care for the musculoskeletal system employ a number of different techniques to condition the body and to help heal injury. The purpose of this section is to give you an idea of the techniques available and the appropriate use of them.

Cold therapy. Common lore recommends application of an ice pack to a newly injured extremity. Experimentally and practically, physicians have found that a cold pack applied immediately to a sprained ligament, an injured joint or a contused muscle will decrease the amount of swelling associated with the injury. The cold must be combined with elevation of the limb and rest for optimal effect. The beneficial effect seems to result from the vasoconstriction (contraction of the blood vessels due to the cold stimulus) and the decrease in metabolic activity. Individuals with arthritis have also found that applying ice to an inflamed joint may help to decrease some of the pain of arthritis. In addition to the direct effect on the tissues, cold compresses have an effect on the nerves, decreasing sensitivity to pain. An ice pack may also be quite helpful in decreasing muscle spasm.

There are some dangers in cold treatments. Individuals with impaired circulation, diabetes, Raynaud's disease or problems with sensation to an extremity should be extremely careful when using cold packs—tissue damage could result.

Hot packs. Heat applied to an extremity can be important in maintaining proper function as well as restoring health to an injured extremity. A limb must be warmed up before any strenuous activity. In cold climates, direct application of a hot pack or other warm object may be most beneficial. When used to treat an injured extremity, heat has proven most helpful for relieving muscle spasms and increasing movement of stiff joints and soft tissues. Heat may be applied in many ways: packs filled with gel (called hydrocalator packs) and immersion in a tub or whirlpool are two other methods. Whirlpool baths are highly touted for their therapeutic effects. Essentially, all types of whirlpools deliver a jet of warm water to a specific part of the body, a treatment almost universally found to be relaxing.

Heat should not be applied to a new injury; it is likely to increase bleeding and swelling. Heat should not be applied to an area of cancer or malignancy, because some studies have shown that growth may be accelerated due to temperature elevations.

Individuals with diabetes or problems with sensation in an extremity must be particularly careful to avoid burns. Application to an inflamed joint may increase the swelling.

Ultrasound. Ultrasound consists of the application of low frequency energy to the body to heat the tissues. It has the advantage of achieving greater depth of penetration than just the application of a hot pack. The absorption of energy, and hence the transmission of heat is related to tissue interfaces, so that ligaments, scar tissue, tendons, capsules of joints and the joint linings tend to absorb more heat with this form of therapy. Ultrasound is particularly useful for the treatment of a condition called myofasciitis, in which the surfaces of the muscles in characteristic locations become quite painful.

13

BRACES FOR THE KNEE

A wide assortment of braces is available for treatment of knee conditions. In simple terms, a brace is a device for restricting the motion of the knee. Bracing is used to protect an unstable knee, to protect a knee while a surgical repair is healing, or to redirect the motion of the kneecap. The degree of restriction of each kind of brace varies.

To understand what a brace is accomplishing, one must consider the normal motion of the knee. The knee normally flexes from 0 degrees (full extension) to approximately 140 degrees (full flexion). While moving, the knee rotates a bit. There is also a limited amount of motion from side to side. During this motion, the patella is supposed to travel smoothly down the center of the groove in the femur. The purpose of a brace is to make sure the motion proceeds in this orderly, controlled fashion. Each kind of brace protects motion in a certain axis. In addition, compression, which is a function of many braces, minimizes swelling. Basically, one can divide the motion of the knee as follows:

1. Flexion and extension
2. Side to side motion
3. Rotation
4. Tracking of the patella

The mechanical effectiveness of many of the very small braces, even those used by professional football players, is mostly overrated. Nevertheless, experience shows that they apparently reduce the number of injuries. This record can be attributed not to the actual ability of the brace to mechanically protect the joint, but rather to a proprioceptive function: The individual is aware of the brace on his knee and perhaps reacts to pressure of the skin against the brace when there is a tendency toward abnormal motion. Laboratory studies do not confirm the effectiveness of many of these types of braces in relieving stress from a knee. No brace will fully control an unstable knee or protect the knee from a massive blow.

The following list categorizes the various types of devices used for protecting the knee:

1. Cast
2. Cast brace
3. Rotation brace
4. Elastic hinge brace
5. Double upright hinge brace
6. Neoprene splint
7. Elastic splint
8. Ace wrap

Cast

A cast provides the maximum amount of joint immobilization: The joint is essentially immobilized in all planes. To truly protect the knee from rotation in a cast, the leg must be bent or flexed. A cast can be made of plaster, as they are traditionally, or some of the new materials such as fiberglass. The disadvantage of the cast, of course, is its bulkiness and the fact that it restricts motion in all planes, leaving the knee rigid. However, immediately following surgery, this degree of immobilization is often necessary.

Cast Brace

A cast brace is similar to a cast except that there are hinges on the side of the knee. A cast brace is highly effective for protecting the knee against forces in a side-to-side plane. Traditionally, cast braces were made out of plaster, but now many commercial firms are manufacturing pre-made braces. One feature of the cast brace is the ability to restrict the range of motion. Following repair of an anterior cruciate ligament, the surgeon may wish to prevent full extension, because straightening the knee will place undue forces across the newly repaired ligament. These restrictions can be built into the hinges of the cast brace.

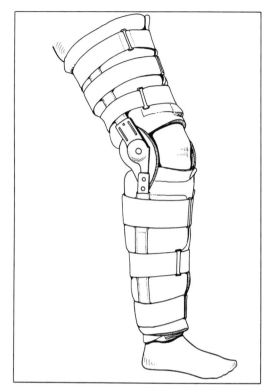

The cast brace is often used for treatment of fractures in the knee area.

The Double Upright Hinge

When there is severe instability of the knee in the side-to-side plane, hinges on each side of the knee may prove adequate for protecting the knee for normal walking. The hinges are often attached to leather which is laced over the thigh and over the leg to stabilize the knee. This type of brace generally does not provide the same rotational control that the cast brace does.

Rotation Brace

This type of brace, developed initially by the brace shop of the Lenox-Hill Hospital in New York City, has been widely used in the United States for protection of knees with rotatory instability. In addition to protecting against side-to-side motion, the brace also can be specially ordered to provide rotational protection. Elastic

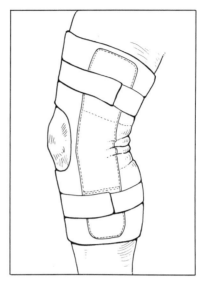

The hinge brace is commonly used by athletes. With an elastic band and two small hinges on the side, it gives stability as well as flexibility.

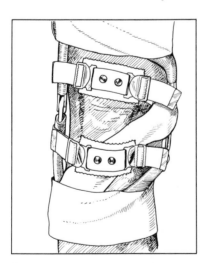

Special braces for control of rotation have been developed by the Lenox-Hill Brace Shop in New York City.

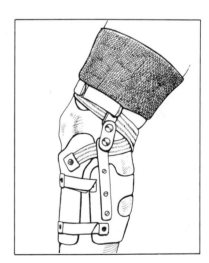

This special brace stabilizes the knee and controls rotation, but it is no substitute for a damaged ligament and is only part of the treatment program.

bands are placed around the leg and, in addition, there are different pressure applicators which tend to resist rotational movements. These braces are commonly used for people who have instability but who are not candidates for surgery and also for additional protection after surgery. In this sense, the brace should be viewed as one part of the treatment of rotatory instability in addition to exercises and activity restrictions. The brace is usually custom-made and requires that the physician make a plaster cast and send it to the brace shop for fitting.

Elastic Hinge Braces

A very popular type of brace, widely available in sports stores, is a hinge contoured on elastic that is applied to the knee. This type is most commonly self-prescribed and used by individuals who feel that their knee is unstable for sports.

This brace provides limited protection from a significant blow to the knee. Experience has shown that many individuals seem to perform at a higher athletic level with the help of this brace and

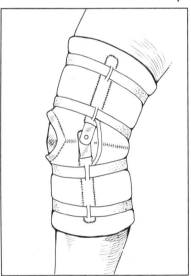

A small-hinge brace seems to reduce the injury rate when used in sports, but it is not mechanically able to prevent injuries.

seem to have few injuries. Much of this improvement is undoubt-edly the proprioceptive function of the brace.

Neoprene Splint

People with patellar problems often find one of the many neo-prene-type splints to be quite helpful. The brace consists of a band of neoprene, usually with a U-shaped piece of felt or similar material underneath the kneecap. The amount of pressure can often be directed individually with small Velcro attachments. This brace can dramatically help someone with patellar problems. It appears to act by slightly redirecting the kneecap medially in

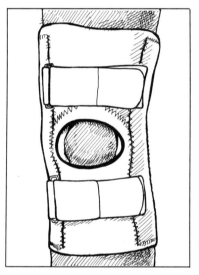

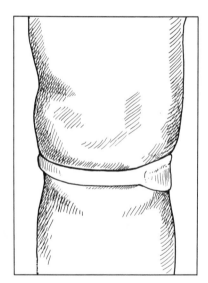

An elastic or neoprene brace, when applied to the knee, may help redirect the motion of the kneecap and decrease patellar pain.

For some people, a small band (Cho-Pat brand shown) wrapped around the knee will decrease the pain associated with some knee-cap problems.

most cases or providing some compressive stability to a lax patellar mechanism.

Elastic Wrap

A very common item available in most sporting goods stores is a cylinder of elastic material for the knee. This device can maintain compression and possibly decrease swelling. It provides virtually no protection other than a proprioceptive function to stabilize the knee.

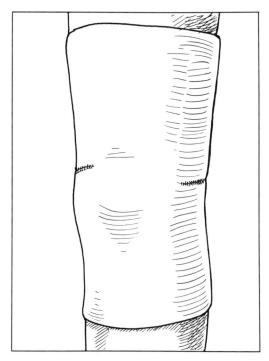

The simplest knee support is an elastic wrap; it has no mechanical function, but may have a minor effect on patellar motion and help reduce swelling.

Ace Wrap

Applying an Ace to the knee may provide some degree of compression for minimizing swelling and may also serve, like the elastic wrap, to stabilize the kneecap. However, it provides absolutely no stability protection.

14

KNEE SURGERY

Recent scientific and medical advances have resulted in knee surgery which is now quite successful in making possible an earlier return to activities and in treating conditions previously considered quite discouraging and virtually inoperable. No operation is undertaken lightly. Surgery involving the knee is generally performed for one of four reasons:

1. Relief of severe pain
2. Restoration of desired function
3. Correction of deformity
4. Prevention of further damage to the joint

For some conditions, an operation is performed only after a prolonged period of more basic treatment such as exercise, physical therapy or arthritis medication. In other situations, orthopedic surgeons know, from their own experience and the research of many scientists and physicians, that if surgery is not performed promptly, the results will not be as good and an unstable or painful knee is very likely to result.

Not all physicians will agree on the indications for an operation or exactly what procedure should be performed, because new techniques and devices are constantly being developed. Successful procedures in the short term do not always continue to provide good function in the long term. Also, many different procedures will produce equally excellent results when performed by a capable surgeon.

Central to any consideration of surgery are the needs and expectations of an individual as well as his state of health. New techniques in anesthesia, infection control, pulmonary physiology, blood banking, surgical materials and many other areas have dramatically decreased the frequency of complications in modern times. Complications, although rare, do occur, and many factors must be considered before deciding on an operation. One must weigh the benefits and advantages of any surgery against the possibility of complications.

CHOOSING YOUR DOCTOR

Selecting a physician to care for your knee problem can be a most frustrating experience. There are no absolute rules for finding the best physician to treat your condition. In our country today, most serious injuries of the extremities are treated by orthopedic surgeons.

An orthopedic surgeon is a specialist in treatment of musculoskeletal problems, including fractures, arthritis and other disturbances of joints. In addition to completing four years of medical school, an orthopedic surgeon receives five additional years of training specifically in surgery and orthopedic surgery. Following successful completion of this training, he can then be called a trained orthopedic surgeon. After practicing orthopedic surgery for two years, a physician may seek certification by an organization called the American Board of Orthopedic Surgery. To be certified by the Board of Orthopedic Surgery, he must successfully complete his orthopedic training in an accredited program. He must also pass a rigorous written and oral examination in which his knowledge of orthopedic surgery and ability to appropriately handle orthopedic problems are evaluated. Following successful completion of the examination, he is then declared to be board-certified. Board certification applies not only to orthopedic surgery; most other specialties have their own individual examinations. There are many fine orthopedic surgeons who are not board-certified, but if you have no prior knowledge of a physician's capabilities, you would be best served by going to a board-certified physician. There is, of course, no absolute guarantee that a particular orthopedic surgeon has extensive experience in treating your kind of problem. However, it gives you some assurance that at some point in his life, the physician passed a rigorous orthopedic examination.

Physicians tend to have good insight into the capabilities of their fellow physicians. Therefore, a good place to start in seeking orthopedic care for your knee is your family physician. He may have referred other patients for orthopedic care and will probably be able to knowledgeably recommend an orthopedic surgeon with experience concerning your type of problem.

In recent times, many physicians have chosen to label themselves as sportsmedicine specialists. Some have received additional training in treatment of athletic-related injuries; others have chosen to concentrate on this area. Such individuals are usually younger than most practicing orthopedic surgeons and have a particular interest in sports injuries. Physicians and scientists who concentrate their research efforts on sports-related injuries have made enormous contributions to the understanding and treatment of knee injuries. Your choice of a physician should be based on his experience and reputation, not just whether he concentrates on sports injuries. In many cases, the broader experience of an orthopedic surgeon who treats not only athletic injuries, but more general musculoskeletal problems as well, may be an advantage to you.

A serious injury to the knee usually requires continuing care. You are going to be dealing with a physician for a long period of time, so he should be someone to whom you can relate, who is sensitive to your individual needs, and who is knowledgeable about your unique requirements. Such a physician should be interested in knowing what demands you plan to make on your knee and what sort of work you do, so the two of you can together establish appropriate treatment. He should be someone willing to take the time to explain in detail the nature of your particular problem and what treatment options are available. If surgery is advised, he should explain the benefits and complications of that particular operation. For some types of conditions, a physician who expresses a desire to work with you to see if non-operative techniques may work may be preferable to one who wishes to perform surgery immediately. For other conditions, most physicians will recommend that early surgery is more likely to yield the best results.

It is perfectly acceptable to ask your physician, when he proposes a certain operation, how many he has done before, what his experience has been, and what complications he has had. A surgeon need not do thousands of a particular operation, but he should have some experience in dealing with your type of problem. One particularly good question to ask a physician who has suggested surgery is about the post-surgical rehabilitation program which he uses. A physician with extensive experience in a procedure should have developed a well thought-out and fairly detailed rehabilitation program. It is indicative of an entire treatment program, including the operation; the actual surgery for a knee injury is only a small part of the entire program necessary for recovery.

ARTHROSCOPY

Arthroscopy represents one of the major recent advances in knee surgery. An arthroscope is a small periscope-like device, often only 1/8 inch in diameter, which can be inserted into the joint.

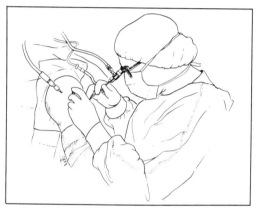

During arthroscopy a surgeon visualizes the inside of the knee. Fiber optics are used to direct light into the knee.

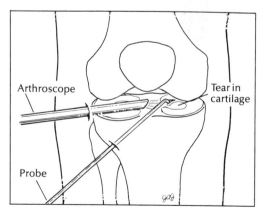

In this arthroscopic surgery, a probe is passed into the knee through another small hole, where it rests in the middle of a tear of the medial meniscus.

Because the device is so small, it is possible for the surgeon to see virtually everywhere in the knee. Studies have shown that this technique can be almost 100 percent accurate in diagnosing cartilage tears.

In some cases, the picture from the arthroscope can be projected onto a television screen. Technology has developed color television cameras approximately the size of a baseball which can be sterilized. These cameras use advanced microelectronic techniques. The surgery may be performed using general or local anesthesia, depending on the clinical situation and an individual's desire. Arthroscopy became popular in the United States in the late 1970s. More than 200,000 arthroscopies are now performed each year. Their popularity has enabled orthopedic surgeons to diagnose knee problems much more accurately and to treat them more promptly and appropriately. Arthroscopy is not a necessary technique for all knee injuries, and a good orthopedic surgeon, of course, only uses it sparingly when he judges it appropriate. A painful knee is not necessarily an indication for you to rush in and have an arthroscopy.

Arthroscopic Surgery

Once a problem has been identified during diagnostic arthroscopy, it is often possible to perform surgery right through the arthroscope, using special micro-instruments. These instruments can be inserted through a channel in the arthroscope in some cases or through a separate small hole elsewhere in the knee. Removal of loose bodies and torn cartilage and shaving of rough surfaces may be done using arthroscopic surgery techniques. Arthroscopic surgery eliminates the traditionally large surgical scar and affords a much faster recovery and return to normal or athletic activities. There is less chance of an infection, and the evidence seems to indicate that there are fewer complications following this surgery. In a subsequent section, the events surrounding an arthroscopic surgical procedure are described in detail.

Arthroscopic Surgery for a Torn Cartilage

The major problem for which arthroscopic surgery is used is treatment of a torn cartilage. These tears may take many forms, as described in the section on Injuries of the Cartilage. In the example shown here, the tear is first visualized through the arthroscope. A small probe with a hook on the end of it is then passed

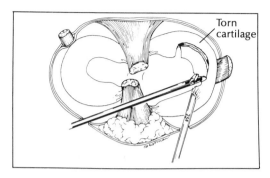

*The surgeon uses the arthroscope and a small
punch to remove a torn portion of cartilage.*

into the knee through a separate small hole, and the tear is outlined to establish the extent of the damage. An instrument called
a basket forceps is then used to remove only the damaged portion of the cartilage. The small particles cut away are taken out
through a separate tubing. Special knives are also used to cut the
cartilage and smooth it down. In some cases, more extensive removal of cartilage may be required, and a micro-shaver is inserted
in the knee. This instrument has a rotating blade, which smooths
down or shaves the torn cartilage. In certain cases the tear in the
cartilage can be repaired. Arthroscopic surgery for meniscal tears
has enabled surgeons to preserve as much cartilage as possible.
Ideally, the mechanics of the knee will be preserved and the likelihood of degenerative arthritis will be decreased.

Arthroscopic Shaving of the Joint Surface

Where the joint surface has been damaged and contains rough
pieces of cartilage, smoothing of the surface may prove quite
beneficial. Smoothing is accomplished by use of micro-instruments and, in many cases, the use of an electric shaver. There is
some early evidence that perhaps roughening or drilling of the
bone down to the level of small blood vessels may enhance the
body's ability to provide a kind of fibrocartilage—an inferior
brand of cartilage, but nevertheless a smooth surface—in areas
where the joint has been eroded down to bone.

Removal of Loose Bodies

Chunks of cartilage and bone may break off and float freely in
the knee. An individual with this problem may experience sudden excruciating pain or the knee may lock or give out. These

loose bodies may be visualized through an arthroscope and, using a special micro-grabber, they can be removed through a separate hole.

ARTHROTOMY

An arthrotomy literally means the opening of a joint. In many cases, an incision into the knee joint is necessary to determine the extent of the disease or injury. Repair of the cruciate ligaments, reattachment of the meniscus, and other extensive reconstruction generally requires that the joint be opened.

Repair of a Meniscus

For many years orthopedic surgeons felt that the meniscus was incapable of repairing itself. Whenever there was a tear in the meniscus, the entire meniscus was removed. There is now some evidence that tears of the meniscus near the edge of the cartilage (where there is adequate blood supply) will heal if held in place. In some instances, sutures are placed across the tear, holding the cartilage in place, and the knee is then placed in a cast until the cartilage can heal. This procedure is a newly developing area and, in the future, advances will undoubtedly be made in this technique.

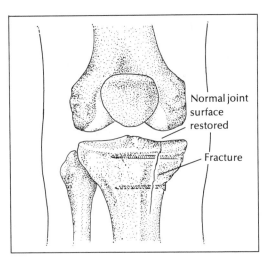

Screws placed across the fracture have, in this case, restored the normal joint surface. There will be less likelihood of arthritis developing from an uneven surface.

Open Reduction and Internal Fixation of Fractures

When a fracture involves the joint surface, it is important that the fragments be put back in place correctly. If the damage to the joint is excessive or if the smooth joint surface cannot be restored, the uneven edges of the damaged joint may result in arthritis. When the fracture involves the growth plate in children, it is vitally important that the architecture of the bone and joint be restored to normal to decrease the chance that disturbance of growth will occur. In the example shown, the fractured kneecap is positioned precisely as before the break and fixed in place with pins.

TREATMENT OF THE TORN ANTERIOR CRUCIATE LIGAMENT

Treatment of the torn anterior cruciate ligament remains one of the most controversial areas of orthopedic surgery. In the past, surgical treatment was discouraging due to unpredictable results, and many individuals, despite an extensive surgical procedure, were not able to return to vigorous activities.

The anterior cruciate ligament has a precarious blood supply and as a result, despite sewing the torn ends back together, in many cases the ligament does not survive. When the ligament is torn in the middle, surgeons generally consider the blood supply to be permanently interrupted and often do not even attempt repair. If the anterior cruciate ligament is damaged and if the knee is unstable, surgery may be necessary to restore stability. It should be emphasized that not everyone with a torn cruciate ligament requires surgery.

Even though surgeons refer specifically to the repair or replacement of the anterior cruciate ligament, the real purpose of the surgery is the restoration of stability with the anterior cruciate playing the lead role in this effort.

The factors which affect the decision to perform surgery were discussed in the "Problems of Ligaments" chapter. In the chronic situation, surgery is generally performed only after a long period of trial rehabilitation, often supplemented with a brace.

The surgeon must first identify the nature of the knee instability associated with the anterior cruciate ligament tear. This analysis makes an important difference in the type of surgery performed. More than 25 different operations have been described for repair of the anterior cruciate ligament and an equal number for treatment of the various instabilities. The surgeon, based on his own personal experience, supplemented by recent research data, a knowledge of the specific injury, and the expectations and demands, must select an appropriate surgical procedure.

Surgery can be divided into four classes:

1. primary repair of the ligament
2. intra-articular repair (in the joint)
3. extra-articular repair (outside of the joint)
4. artificial ligament

Primary Repair of the Ligament

In cases where the ligament has been torn from bone, repair may be successful. Drill holes are made in the bone, and sutures which are attached to the torn ligament are threaded through the holes.

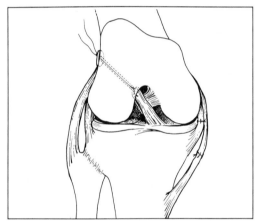

In this case the anterior cruciate ligament has been pulled from the bone; it is reattached by drilling a hole through the bone and threading a suture through it. The medial collateral ligament is also sewn back together.

Intra-Articular Repair

In this technique, tendons from around the knee are transferred into the knee joint to take the place of the anterior cruciate ligament. The hamstrings are a frequent source as is the iliotibial band. One popular technique uses a strip of the patellar tendon which is twisted backwards into the knee and placed into two holes drilled into appropriate places in the tibia and femur.

There is still concern about the lack of blood supply to the tendon, which is responsible for a certain number of failures.

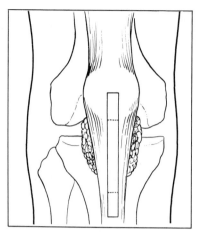

One popular and effective operation for a torn anterior cruciate ligament is a transfer of a portion of
the patellar tendon to take the
place of the irreparably damaged
anterior cruciate ligament.

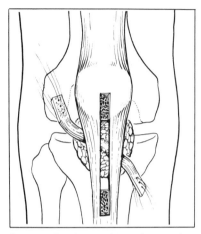

In a tendon transplant, the tendon
is removed from its normal site in
the patella with the attached fat
and blood supply and transferred
back into the area of the cruciate
ligament.

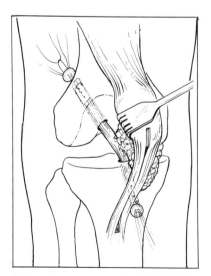

Following placement of drill holes
at the sites where the damaged anterior cruciate ligament was attached, the new tendon is transferred and secured in place with
sutures.

Extra-Articular Repair

The third alternative method of repair is to use tendons and ligaments that run on the outside of the knee joint and reroute or transfer them to imitate the function of the anterior cruciate ligament. Taking a part of the iliotibial band and moving it to tighten the structures on the outside of the knee, preventing the tibia from being pulled forward, is one example. The so-called "pes plasty," in which the tendons of the pes anserinus are transferred, is another way in which the direction of the muscle pull is changed to promote stability.

The Torn Medial Collateral Ligament

In most cases, an isolated tear of the medial collateral ligament is treated in a cast followed by a cast brace. In cases where surgery is indicated, the ends of the torn ligament are approximated and sutures placed across the torn ends to hold them in position. In some cases, where there has been extensive damage to the capsule and the medial collateral ligament, a group of tendons called the pes anserinus is transferred to reinforce the repair of the damaged structures. The capsule at the inside of the knee in back is also repaired during this procedure.

Repair of the Posterior Cruciate Ligament

The posterior cruciate ligament lies primarily at the back of the knee. A functional posterior cruciate ligament is essential for normal knee function. In many cases, the ligament is pulled off from the tibia with a piece of bone attached. If this bone is pulled away, it is put back where it belongs and a screw placed across to hold it in the correct position. The leg is then placed in a cast until this bone heals. In cases where the posterior cruciate ligament is irreparably damaged, other tendons and muscles may be transferred to restore stability. Often, however, an appropriate exercise program is successful treatment for a torn posterior cruciate ligament, and surgery is not necessary.

Artificial Anterior Cruciate Ligaments

Considerable research is being conducted to develop an acceptable artificial ligament. The requirements of the knee are quite demanding:

1) It must be strong—about 125 pounds of force are placed across the cruciate ligament during normal walking. The normal anterior cruciate ligament in a young adult can withstand 450 pounds of force.

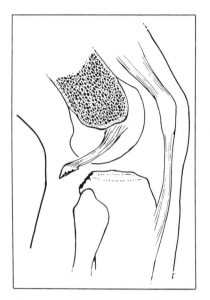

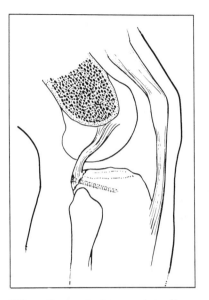

The posterior cruciate ligament may be ripped from its attachment along with a piece of bone.

When the posterior cruciate ligament is attached to a large piece of bone, the bone is held in place and secured with a special bone screw.

2) It must bend easily—the ligament is pulled in a circular motion with every step. An artificial ligament must be not only strong but pliable.

3) It must not cause rejection—an artificial ligament is a foreign substance and must be made of a material which does not stimulate the body's immune system and cause an inflammatory response.

4) It must not wear out—an average person takes more than 10 million steps in a lifetime. A successful replacement for the ligament must be able to withstand this punishment.

5) It must not stretch out—the normal cruciate ligament has a relatively constant resiliency, known to scientists as a modulus of elasticity. A replacement must have a similar mechanical property.

An artificial ligament is used for two reasons: (1) to stabilize the knee while one's own ligament or a transferred ligament gains enough strength to support the knee; and (2) to completely replace an irreparably torn ligament. In this latter case, an artificial ligament is currently only used as a last resort, when one's own supporting structures have failed.

Artificial ligaments are of two types: synthetic and biological. They are also divided into two classifications based on their adaptation to the body: biodegradable and permanent.

The different materials currently being tested include Dacron, polypropylene, bovine tendon and carbon fibers. Research scientists at many different centers are performing experiments in animals and controlled studies in humans to develop an acceptable artificial ligament. To date, no adequate artificial replacement for the anterior cruciate ligament has been developed, although some replacements have proven sufficient for temporary protection.

SURGERY FOR KNEECAP ALIGNMENT PROBLEMS

A kneecap which does not travel in the proper direction and continues to cause pain or dislocate despite exhaustive exercises may require surgical redirection.

There are basically three types of surgery for this condition. In the first type, the place where the patellar tendon attaches to the bone is moved, so the kneecap is directed more toward the inside of the knee. In the second type, the fibers attached to the outside or lateral side of the kneecap are released, allowing travel medially. In the third type, the muscles attached to the top of the kneecap are re-attached so they pull more toward the inside.

Each of these procedures has advantages and disadvantages, and all may prove successful. The procedure chosen depends on your individual problem and the experience of your surgeon.

The Lateral Release

The kneecap may be tilted to the outside, resulting in uneven pressure. Surgical release of the fibers on the lateral side of the kneecap (lateral retinaculum) and of the muscle that pulls the kneecap laterally (vastus lateralis) will, in many cases, allow normal motion of the knee. This procedure has the advantage of not requiring a cast following surgery.

Patellar Realignment by Muscle Transfer

In some individuals, the patella is pulled so much to the outside that mere lateral release of the tissues on the side of the kneecap is inadequate. To change the course of motion of the patella and relieve the uneven pressure, the muscles on the inside of the knee are transferred to a point near the middle of the kneecap to pull the kneecap more medially toward the inside.

Patellar Tendon Transfer

Treatment of a repeatedly dislocating kneecap may require extensive surgery. One technique is to transfer the point where the patellar tendon connects to the front of the tibia: removing a piece of bone from the tibia, moving it to the inside, and placing a screw into the bone to hold it in place.

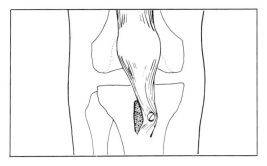

Some people are born with a kneecap that is pulled to the outside. To achieve proper alignment of the kneecap in front of the knee, surgery may be required. The patellar tendon, along with its bony attachment on the tibia, is moved to a new position and screwed in place.

Patellar Shaving

The kneecap may become unevenly worn and have areas of exposed bone or irregular cartilage. These areas may look like cotton or seaweed. Smoothing of the roughened areas may help relieve pain. Drilling holes into the exposed bone may also encourage fibrocartilage to form on the undersurface of the kneecap. Where the kneecap is now aligned or tilted, realignment may also be necessary.

New Cartilage for Old Joints

The idea of transplanting cartilage to take the place of a worn-out joint has intrigued scientists for many years. A very substantial research effort has been devoted to this task, starting with experimental animals and progressing to pioneering work with humans. Part of this intense interest has been recognition of the

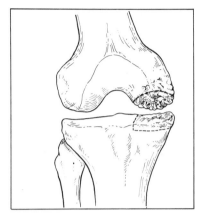

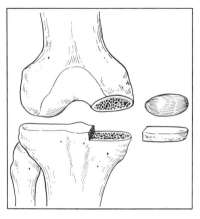

The damaged cartilage shown is removed and the site prepared for implantation of new cartilage.

A cadaver serves as a cartilage donor. The site of the joint which is needed is removed from a matched donor.

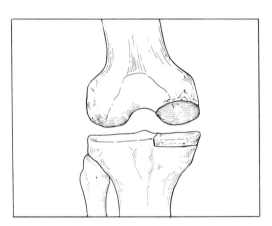

Following removal of the donor cartilage, the cartilage is implanted in the recipient and held firmly in place.

limitations of artificial joints, which, although quite successful, are prone to loosening, infection and mechanical failure. Currently, at a few university centers in select cases, physicians are replacing parts of joints and even whole segments of bone and joint with matching parts from a suitable donor.

Unfortunately, the human body has a very limited supply of extra cartilage which can be transplanted from one joint to another. Thus, scientists have been forced to depend upon transplants from a deceased person. Cartilage depends upon the synovial fluid of the joint for nutrition, so unlike bone, it does not need a new blood supply. When intact cartilage is transplanted with only a small rim of bone, rejection by the immunologic system of the recipient does not seem to be an insurmountable problem.

Experience in human beings so far is limited but promising. Transplants have sometimes consisted of whole segments of bone and joints in cases where the operation was performed to replace tissue destroyed by malignant tumor. In other cases, only an isolated area of destroyed cartilage was replaced. When large segments of bone are included, problems of rejection, fracture, infection, and failure to heal are particularly worrisome.

Transplantation of isolated areas of a joint depends upon a precise fit of the parts if the cartilage is to endure the repetitive stress of a normal joint for an extended period of time. In practical terms, the donor's joint must be a near-perfect match to the recipient's. Furthermore, to maximize the chances of survival of the cartilage cells, transplantation must be accomplished within 12 to 24 hours. Many details of selection, storage and surgical technique must be perfected before this procedure becomes a reality on a large scale. However, there is every reason to believe that transplantation of cartilage will be a valuable tool for the treatment of certain arthritic disorders.

15

ARTHROSCOPY

Prior to undergoing an arthroscopy, you will have a pre-operative evaluation by your family physician and your orthopedic surgeon. For a young healthy individual, this procedure is simple and straightforward. For someone with multiple medical problems, a more thorough evaluation may be required, generally including some simple blood tests and a urinalysis. If there is an indication of other medical problems, a more extensive laboratory evaluation will be performed.

The Night Before Surgery

On the evening prior to your surgery, you will be advised not to have anything to eat or drink after midnight. This rule includes any coffee, soft drinks or even water. This precaution is recommended because during the anesthesia, there is the possibility of vomiting. If it occurs, fluid could get into the lungs and cause serious pneumonia. Therefore, before any elective surgery, precautions are taken so that there is no food or fluid in the stomach.

Arrival for Surgery

All arthroscopic surgery is performed in a sterile operating room. In most cases, general anesthesia is used. In many communities there are surgery centers—separate health care facilities devoted to outpatient surgery. In other areas, surgery is performed in a hospital, but on an outpatient basis: You come in to the hospital, have the surgery done, and go home the same day.

When arriving for surgery, you will be questioned regarding your name, your surgeon's name, and which leg is to be operated on. A name band will be placed around your wrist so you will be properly identified in case of an unanticipated emergency. These details may seem somewhat repetitious, but they are important to prevent any errors.

The Changing Room

You will be shown into a changing room where your clothes will be checked and you will change into a hospital gown. Then you will be shown into an area of the hospital called the holding room. In the holding room, once again you will be questioned regarding your name, your physician, and which leg is to undergo surgery. In addition, the area around your knee will be shaved so hair will not get in the way of the surgery. In times past, this shaving was sometimes done the evening before, but studies have shown that there is less likelihood of infection if it is done immediately prior to surgery. An intravenous line will be started to supply a route for the administration of medication.

The Anesthesia Interview

If you are going to have general anesthesia, an anesthesiologist will interview you prior to the surgery. He will inquire about any problems with previous surgery and any drug allergies. He will be specifically interested in knowing if any members of your family have had problems with surgery or anesthesia. This information is important because some very serious reactions to anesthesia tend to run in families. Following this interview, the anesthesiologist will prescribe an injection called a pre-med: a drug to dry your secretions and, in most cases, a narcotic to help you relax. You may note that your vision is slightly blurred following the injection, but this should not worry you.

The Operating Room

Following these preparations, you will be taken on a stretcher to the operating room suite itself—a special room only used for surgery. Everyone in the room wears a sterile gown, booties, a hair cover, and a mask. The room has a specially filtered air system to eliminate dust and contamination. You will be moved from the stretcher to the operating table, and monitoring electrodes will be attached with small sticky discs. These are connected to a monitor which indicates your pulse and the electrical activity of your heart. In addition, a blood pressure cuff will be placed around your arm so that your blood pressure can be taken at regular intervals during the course of the operation.

The Operating Room Team

The operating team is a highly trained group of individuals who rigorously adhere to the standards required for surgery. That is one of the reasons why there are relatively few surgical complications in the United States. You will have previously met the anesthesiologist who spoke with you in the holding room. In some cases, a nurse-anesthetist will assist him during part of the procedure. The scrub nurse, prior to your arrival in the room, has scrubbed her hands and arms and is now gowned in a sterile gown and gloves. She is responsible for handling sterile instruments and for assisting the surgeon during the performance of the arthroscopy. The circulating nurse, who is also present in the room, is responsible for the direction of the room. She is always a registered (R.N.) nurse, and it is her responsibility to ensure that the correct patient has the correct operation performed. She will check your armband to be sure you're the right person, will also inquire again as to your name, your physician, and the leg to be operated upon. She may go in and out of the room during the surgery to obtain necessary supplies.

Beginning of Surgery

Prior to administering an anesthetic, the anesthesiologist will check your vital signs (pulse and blood pressure). If all are normal, the anesthetic agent will be administered. In most cases, pentathol, or some variation, will be given through the intravenous line already started. A mask will be placed over your nose and mouth, and gases, known as inhalation agents, will also be given. Oxygen is also administered through this mask. In some cases, when the surgery will be lengthy, a tube, called an endotracheal tube, will be passed through your mouth down into the trachea. This tube provides a direct route for the gases to pass from the anesthesia machine directly into your lungs without any chance of escaping. This procedure provides a degree of safety, but one of the side effects is that you may wake up with hoarseness and a slight sore throat which should pass in a day or so. Following administration of the anesthesia, the anesthesiologist will indicate to the surgeon when it is safe to go ahead with the operation.

Preparation for the Operation

In most cases, a tourniquet similar to a blood pressure cuff is placed around the leg. If necessary, this tourniquet is used to temporarily interrupt the blood supply to the leg. Particularly if extensive work is to be done, the tourniquet facilitates successful surgery by keeping blood away from the operative site. The knee also generally is placed in a leg holder which positions it solidly on the operating room table.

The Prep

The knee is then held by an assistant, and an iodine containing solution is applied to the leg to sterilize the skin. Sterile drapes are then wrapped around the leg to insure the sterility of the operation.

The Operation

The knee is filled with fluid through a small hole and tube. In most cases, saline (a salt solution) is used. The arthroscope is then inserted in the knee and the surgeon can visualize the contents of the knee. The surgeon may look directly into the arthroscope, or in many operating rooms, a very small television camera is used and the image of the contents of the knee is displayed on a television screen. The surgeon thoroughly evaluates the inside of the knee to determine the cause of your problem. In most cases, a separate small instrument is passed into another small hole, allowing the surgeon to lift up the cartilages or to grab loose bodies in the knee.

Arthroscopic Instruments

A whole new generation of instruments has been developed for arthroscopic surgery. The color television camera itself is approximately the size of a baseball and fits right on the end of the arthroscope. The instruments inserted into the knee are about one-eighth of an inch in diameter and enable the surgeon to cut portions of torn menisci, to punch out defects, to remove loose bodies, and to shave uneven surfaces of cartilage.

Removing a Torn Cartilage

The surgeon passes a micro-instrument called a probe into the knee to outline the extent of the tear. He then chooses the appropriate instrument for removal of the torn part of the cartilage, if removal is necessary.

The Dressing

Following completion of the surgery, a sterile dressing is applied to the knee. A compressive Ace wrap is then applied to the leg to decrease the swelling and provide some protection against developing inflammation of the veins of the calf.

Post-Operative Course

After the surgery is completed, you are placed on a stretcher and taken to a special room called the recovery room. In the recovery room, monitors are once again connected, and a nurse closely monitors your recovery. Your blood pressure and your pulse are taken on a regular interval until you have awakened. When adequately awake, you will sit up in a chair and crutches will be provided. In some cases, the crutches will have been fitted prior to the surgery.

Home

Once certain that you are sufficiently recovered from the surgery, you will be discharged from the surgery center or hospital. An instruction sheet will be provided to alert you regarding any complications.

POST-OPERATIVE INFORMATION FOR ARTHROSCOPIC SURGERY

Description

The operation you have just completed consisted of insertion of an arthroscope into the knee to visualize the contents of the knee and diagnose your problem. The knee was filled with fluid through a separate, small hole. Surgery, if necessary, has been performed using special micro-instruments.

Dressing

A bulky, soft dressing has been applied to your knee and held firmly in place with a compressive Ace wrap. The dressing typically has some fluid and blood on it. Two days after the surgery, you may remove this dressing and apply Band-Aids to each of the small holes. If the dressing feels too tight, remove the Ace and re-wrap it to alleviate the pressure. In most cases, there will be three small holes which have been used to perform the arthroscopic surgery. There may be some mild bruising of the skin as well as some swelling, but these symptoms should not be alarming.

Pain

A prescription for pain medication has been written for you consisting of acetaminophen (Tylenol) with codeine, unless you have problems with this medication. You should take one to two tablets every three hours. If you develop any problem with the drug, call the office. The application of an ice pack to the knee may help relieve the pain and reduce the swelling.

Bathing

Do not get your knee wet until I have had a chance to examine it.

Activity

You will almost certainly need crutches for the first few days following surgery. If more complex surgery has been performed, the knee may be more painful and require support for longer periods of time. You may step down on the leg at any time, but be sure control of the leg has been regained before you get rid of the support. Crutches may be completely discarded if the pain decreases and your strength increases.

Exercises

Gentle exercises should be started soon after surgery. The amount of exercise performed will be a function of the pain. You should exercise to your tolerance. On the day of your surgery, you should practice stretching the quadriceps muscle, the muscle on the front of the thigh. Then proceed to straight leg raising. At least 15 minutes each day should be devoted to exercising. Muscles tend to atrophy or waste away quickly if not used. You must work diligently to achieve a rapid recovery.

Problems

If you develop a fever of 101 degrees F. or above, with severe pain, redness, swelling of the calf or any other alarming problem, please call the office. If I am not in the office, the answering service can locate me or my partner immediately if there is an emergency.

Office Appointments

You will need to be seen in the office approximately one week following the surgery. At that time you will be examined, and the details of your particular exercise program will be outlined.

Bending Your Knee

You may bend your knee as much as it is comfortable and tolerated. This exercise should not be forceful or excessively painful.

Meals

Your first meal at home should be clear liquids to avoid getting nauseated following the anesthesia.

Positioning the Knee

On the night following surgery, elevating the knee will help reduce swelling. An ice bag may decrease pain. Do not place a pillow under your knee.

Increasing Activities

Pain should be a guide to activity level. Too much pain indicates too much activity. Do not engage in any sports, running, squatting or twisting. Do not use any exercise machines until I have discussed their use with you.

16

TOTAL KNEE REPLACEMENT

Destruction of the articular cartilage of the knee may be so severe, the arthritis so crippling and painful, that it is necessary to replace the entire knee joint. Approximately 70,000 total knee replacements are performed each year in the United States. This procedure relieves severe pain which has not responded to effective medical management, provides motion and stability to the knee, and corrects disabling deformity. An individual's health and level of activity as well as his expectations for the surgery must be considered carefully to determine whether the risk associated with the operation is appropriate. Persons with poor health, no sensation in the joint, active infection, or severe loss of calcium (osteoporosis) from their bones should not undergo such an operation.

The surgical procedure starts with removal of the worn-out bone and cartilage from the surface of the joint. The joint often has been worn out in an irregular fashion so that the patient is either severely knock-kneed or bow-legged. This deformity must be corrected. The bones are then lined up so that the forces will be evenly distributed, and the components cemented in place using a substance called methylmethacrylate. (Some new replacements do not require cement.) Research continues to develop new metals, new plastics and polyethylene materials which are more durable for the very demanding needs of a total knee replacement.

The operation will not succeed without the active involvement of the patient following surgery. It takes a great deal of patience, hard work and sacrifice to achieve a good result.

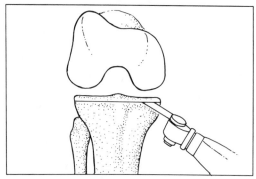

To remove an old tibial joint, the tibial plateau is carefully removed so that the new joint may be placed on a flat surface.

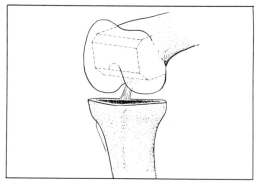

To replace a worn-out femoral joint, the surface of the femur is removed using a saw so that a new metallic knee may be put in place.

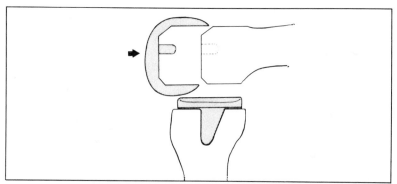

After cutting the femur and gluing in a new knee component on the top of the flattened tibia, the metal femoral component of the new knee is placed on the end of the bone.

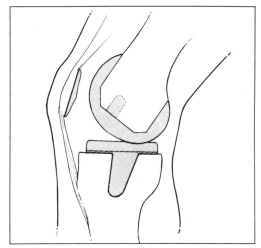

*The total knee replacement consists of a patel-
lar button cemented on the back of the kneecap, a metal shell that fits on the end of the femur and a polyethylene surface that is
cemented on top of the tibia.*

Complications Following Total Knee Replacement

Although the surgeon takes extraordinary precautions, complications can and do occur with surgery. Special measures are
taken to prevent complications. Antibiotics are given to every patient who undergoes total knee replacement to decrease the possibility of infection. Suction drainage is used to carry away any
blood that may collect and could cause problems in the new
knee. Special elastic stockings are worn by all patients to decrease the chances of developing blood clots in the legs. A special breathing device, an incentive spirometer, is used by each patient to keep the lungs functioning well and to prevent possible
collapse of small air sacs or development of pneumonia. Patients
can stand in a special bed developed by the Stryker Corporation
and are allowed up when comfortable, usually by the second day.
Early mobility is one of the most important features of the post-
operative program to restore a person to normal function and decrease the likelihood of many complications.

An infection may occur immediately after an operation, or a total joint replacement may become infected from bacteria found
elsewhere in the body at any time, months or even years following the initial surgery. This problem is one of the most serious
complications of the surgery and may necessitate removal of the
knee replacement. Infections of the knee have been caused by

tooth abscesses, dental manipulation, urinary tract infections or pneumonia. These infections occur when bacteria from another site travel in the blood to the new joint. If an individual develops an infection anywhere in the body, it is extremely important that antibiotics be started immediately.

A small percentage of patients who have total joint replacements will experience loosening of their new joint. The longer a joint is in place, the more likely this loosening is to occur. The knee is not well-protected, and a knee replacement is not intended for someone who is quite active or who wants to play sports. Vigorous activity, trauma and obesity often can loosen a joint. Pain or progressive deformity may necessitate more surgery. Artificial joints are not as sturdy as the real ones and, because they are not made of biologic tissue, cannot repair themselves. The possibility of loosening is one of the primary reasons why joint replacements are not advised for young, vigorous individuals.

The following is a description of the events surrounding a total knee replacement. Certain details may vary from hospital to hospital, but the basic care and precautions should be similar in most established institutions.

Day #1. Two days before surgery, you are seen in the admitting office of the hospital and formally admitted as a patient. Certain basic information is obtained, and a band is placed around your wrist to ensure your identity if you are unconscious. You are then escorted to your room and introduced to the staff who will be caring for you. Each floor has a head nurse, individual registered nurses, licensed practical nurses and nurses' aides, who are present 24 hours a day. The nurse who will be caring for you will ask about specific health problems and your personal needs. The orthopedic surgery house officer will then take a history and perform a physical examination.

Day #2. A dietician from the hospital will interview you, particularly if there is a need for a special diet such as low-salt or diabetic. A physical therapist will assess your current capabilities and demonstrate the demands that will be made after joint replacement. In most cases, some laboratory studies will have been done in advance. These include blood studies, a urine sample, a chest X ray and an electrocardiogram. A culture of the urine will have been done to make sure that there is no infection in the bladder or kidneys. Other, more sophisticated tests may also have been requested for more serious medical problems. Because a blood transfusion is usually necessary, a blood sample will be taken, and a procedure called a "type and cross" will be performed. This test assures that a blood transfusion, if needed during or after your surgery, will match or be compatible with your own blood.

The anesthesiologist will then review your history and interview you regarding the anesthesia for the operation. At this time, you should ask any questions you may have about the anesthesia and explain any problems you may have had with previous operations. You will then be shown a special bed used for this operation called a circle electric bed. This bed was designed by Dr. Homer Stryker of Kalamazoo, Mich. It allows you to stand upright in the bed. The nurses or orthopedic technicians will instruct you in the use of this bed.

Special stockings, called anti-embolism hose, will be fitted to reduce the likelihood of blood clots developing in the calf during the hospitalization. On the evening prior to surgery, you will be advised to have nothing to eat or drink after midnight, referred to in medical terms as NPO. This precaution is necessary so that there will be no fluid or food in the stomach while the anesthesia is being administered. Some people react adversely to the medications and vomit during surgery. If this acidic fluid gets into the lungs, it can cause what is known as an aspiration pneumonia. Severe complications may result.

Day #3. Early in the morning on the day of surgery (sometimes the evening before), an intravenous line will be started. A sterile plastic or metal needle is inserted in a vein in your arm and a salt (saline) and sugar (dextrose) solution is dripped in at a prescribed rate. The purpose of this intravenous line or IV is to furnish a direct route for the administration of medications, particularly antibiotics, and to provide necessary fluids during the operation and right after surgery, when you are not capable of feeding yourself.

Approximately an hour before surgery, you will be given an injection ordered by the anesthesiologist called the " prelim." This shot usually consists of atropine (or a similar drug), a chemical that will dry secretions and may blur your vision, plus another medication to relax you. You are then taken from your room to a room known as the holding room in the operating suite. Upon admission to the holding room, your entire record, including laboratory studies, is reviewed. Blood transfusions are generally required during surgery, so a check is made to be sure the transfusion is ready. As a safeguard, several nurses will ask your name, the operation to be performed, the side to be operated upon (right or left), and the name of your doctor. This information will be checked against the arm band you are wearing. The procedure may seem repetitious, but it is important—vitally so—to avoid a mistake. Once it has been determined that everything is in order, you will be taken by stretcher to the operating room itself and moved onto an operating table.

The operating room is a very special room. There you will meet members of the team who will assist in the performance of your surgery. A successful operation is the result of a coordinated effort by a very devoted, dedicated and highly trained team of surgical and hospital personnel. Each link in the team is vital. Before your arrival in the operating room, a great deal of preparation has been made to ensure all will go well. Special instruments required for a total knee replacement have been checked, sterilized and re-checked after being removed from sterile containers. In addition, the implant to be placed is prepared in multiple sizes to conform to individual differences. Such differences can only be determined during the surgery when the old knee joint is removed. A check has been made to make certain that all necessary components are available for your case. The room has undergone a cleaning for sterility, and only those individuals who are absolutely required to be present are allowed into the room. Operating rooms have special ventilation systems that filter the air to minimize the number of bacteria. All members of the operating team are dressed in special gowns, and all wear hats, masks and booties to prevent the spread of any bacteria from the hair, nose, mouth and shoes.

Special electrodes are placed on your skin, connected to a cardiac monitor to assess your pulse and the electrical activity of your heart during the operation. A blood pressure cuff is placed on one of your arms so your blood pressure can be monitored every few minutes during surgery.

The anesthesiologist who will be administering the anesthesia checks the intravenous line to be sure it is functioning properly. He prepares to administer the anesthesia by checking the availability of all necessary drugs and making certain the anesthesia machine is functioning properly. The anesthesia machine contains many important instruments and gauges, multiple tanks of gas including oxygen, nitrous oxide (laughing gas), fluothane (an anesthetic agent), a small rubber bag that is squeezed to push air into the lungs, and an exhaust hose that carries away any anesthetic substance that may leak.

Medications are given through the fluid line in your vein, and gas anesthesia is usually administered through a mask. First, a process called oxygenation is performed in which you breathe pure oxygen in and out. Following administration of anesthetic medication, a tube called an endotracheal tube is passed through the mouth down into the trachea to make sure that the oxygen and anesthetic gasses go directly to the lungs in a controlled fashion. This procedure also avoids any leakage of fluid into the lungs, either from the stomach or from the mouth. The tube may cause throat irritation for a few days following surgery. All the vital signs such as pulse and blood pressure are reassessed to be sure there has been no adverse reaction to the anesthesia. Some individuals choose to have a spinal anesthetic, in which case a small needle is used to inject the numbing medication into the spinal canal. These individuals can breathe by themselves and do not need respiratory support.

The anesthesiologist then indicates that the operation can proceed. The leg to be operated upon is held in position, and a wide area of skin is scrubbed, usually with an iodine solution, and then painted with another iodine solution to further eliminate any contamination. This preparation is usually performed by the circulating nurse. She is attired in a special surgical scrub suit, but is not wearing a sterile gown. Therefore, she is free to move about in the room to obtain needed supplies and to open special containers containing the sterile implants and instruments. While your skin is being prepared, the surgeon and the assistant surgeon are scrubbing their hands and arms to remove bacterial contamination. Sterile gowns and gloves are then put on. The area about to be operated upon has sterile drapes placed around it to separate it from the rest of your body. You are now ready for the operation.

When surgery is finished, a sterile gauze dressing is placed over the surgical site, and the drain that has been placed deep in the knee is taped to the skin. The purpose of this drain is to siphon out any small amounts of blood that may collect and eliminate it from the body rather than allowing it to collect and cause problems. During the surgery, the anesthesiologist, in consultation with the surgeon, may determine that there has been enough blood loss to justify a transfusion. The transfusion is performed during the operation before there is any problem. A considerable volume of fluid is also administered through the intravenous line during the surgery.

After the operation, you are transferred onto a stretcher or a special circle electric bed and taken to the recovery room. The room is equipped with special monitoring devices and all of the resuscitation equipment necessary, should there be any problems following surgery. A registered nurse will again monitor your vital signs very closely and administer pain medication as necessary. You will be groggy for many hours after surgery and will probably have only a sketchy recollection of the events that took place. You will remain in the recovery room for an hour or two until the supervising anesthesiologist is sure you are stable and ready to be transferred back to your room. Meanwhile, the surgeon meets your family in the waiting room to discuss the surgery.

Following return to your hospital room, your condition will be closely monitored around the clock by your nurses. Orders for your care have been written by the surgeon. Everyone has pain following surgery, and specific orders have been given regarding the administration of pain medications. Generally, you will require narcotic injections for the first day or two.

Day #4 (First Post-operative Day). The first post-operative day is probably the roughest day of the whole experience. There will still be considerable pain, and you will probably still require injections for relief. The intravenous line is kept running and fluids are administered, because most individuals have still not recovered enough to eat normally. Antibiotics are given for the first 48 hours to decrease the chance of developing an infection. Laboratory samples are taken in the morning. A blood sample will determine your fluid status and show if there has been any change in your blood count. If there has been continued blood loss, a blood transfusion may be given.

One particular complication after surgery is the development of pneumonia and collapse of the small sacs in the lungs. For this reason, all patients undergoing total knee surgery receive instruction in the use of a special device called an inspirometer. Some people have difficulty urinating due to all the pain medication and the fact that they are lying in bed; a catheter tube may have to be placed directly into the bladder through the urethra. Attempts are made to avoid this procedure, but sometimes it is necessary. In addition to the laboratory studies, measurements are made concerning the amount of fluid which flows in through the intravenous line and the amount that is excreted as well as the precise amount of drainage found in the drain. Your blood pressure, pulse and temperature will be taken every four hours and more frequently if there are any abnormalities.

The circle bed will allow you to stand while remaining in bed, even on the first day after the surgery. You will probably not be very hungry and will be given just a liquid diet during this first day.

Day #5 (Second Post-operative Day). The post-surgical pain should be considerably less by the second day, and many find that they are able to take pain pills rather than receive injections. Another blood sample will be drawn in the morning to determine the status of your electrolytes and your red blood cells. If everything is in order, and if you are consuming an adequate amount of fluids, the intravenous line will be removed. The drain is then pulled out and the dressing over the surgical site is changed. If you are feeling well enough, you may be allowed to take a few steps at this time—only if accompanied by the nurses.

Day #6 (Third Post-operative Day). On this day you should be recovering some of your strength and will begin to take a few more steps in your room. You will go to the physical therapy department to begin relearning control of the involved limb as well as use of a walker or crutches. A special plan of therapy is followed for patients who have had a total knee replacement. You will begin relying considerably on the physical therapist for support while walking with the use of parallel bars. Special strengthening exercises will also be performed to aid in recovery. While in your room, your vital signs will continue to be monitored closely.

Day #7. In general, you will go to the physical therapy department twice a day to continue exercises and learn to use walking aids. Generally, by this time you will have advanced to the use of a walker or, in some cases, crutches. More exercises will be performed at each physical therapy session.

Day #8 to Discharge. Physical therapy is continued daily. Your strength and endurance should be increasing. During the week, you will be seen by an occupational therapist, who will assess your skills and provide counseling so that you can adapt to this new situation. Devices such as long-arm reachers will be furnished to assist you in picking up things from the floor and in reaching—a necessary precaution to avoid undue strain. From this time until your discharge from the hospital, therapy will be continued to increase your strength, coordination and agility. You will receive instruction in stair climbing and getting in and out of a chair or car. After discharge from the hospital, arrangements will be made for your care to continue in the surgeon's office where the stitches will be removed. You will also receive a prescription for pain medication to be taken at home. Most importantly, you will be cautioned to contact the surgeon should any problems develop.

INDEX

ABOUT THE AUTHOR

Alan A. Halpern, M.D., is a board-certified Orthopedic surgeon practicing in Kalamazoo, Mich. He is a clinical instructor in the department of surgery, Michigan State University College of Human Medicine. He received his orthopedic training at Stanford University and his doctor of medicine degree at Yale University. He has written numerous research articles in the medical literature and is the author of The Kalamazoo Arthritis Book.